Revision Guide for MRCPsych Paper B

This text covers the key information necessary to pass Paper B of the postgraduate examination and become a member of the Royal College of Psychiatrists (MRCPsych).

It provides candidates with comprehensive coverage of the Paper B syllabus, including information from a wide variety of sources to save candidates crucial time during exam revision. The content is accessible and presented in manageable sections, highlighting key information using tables, lists and graphics.

This text is essential for psychiatry trainees revising for their written examinations and is also suitable for individuals/healthcare professionals with an interest in psychiatry and a desire to learn more.

Arun Arujun Bhaskaran, MBBS, BSc (Hons), MRCPsych, graduated from King's College London and completed his foundation training in Ipswich. He then went to complete his core psychiatry training in North Central London and is now a specialist registrar in child and adolescent psychiatry working for the North East London Foundation Trust, UK. Dr Bhaskaran has a keen interest in medical education and completed a postgraduate certificate in medical education during his core training. Throughout his career, he has been regularly involved in training foundation doctors and undergraduates.

Elijah Casper-Blake, MBBS, BSc (Hons), MRCPsych, graduated from Barts and the London School of Medicine and Dentistry. He completed his foundation training in the South Thames Deanery and undertook core psychiatry training in North Central London. Currently, he is working as a specialist registrar in East London, UK. Alongside his work with older adults, Dr Elijah Casper-Blake has a particular interest in substances misuse. Over the course of his career, Dr Elijah Casper-Blake has been involved in training both medical students and fellow doctors.

Richard William Kerslake, MBBS, MRCPsych, is a consultant psychiatrist in older persons' psychiatry. He is a graduate of Royal Free and University College London Medical School. Dr Kerslake is currently working in Sussex, having previously worked and trained in London and Melbourne. He is an honorary clinical lecturer at Brighton & Sussex Medical School, UK, where he is proud to lead the psychiatry rotations for physician associate students, whilst passionately maintaining teaching commitments through lecturing and simulation-based education.

Revision Guide for MRCPsych Paper B

Arun Arujun Bhaskaran,
Elijah Casper-Blake, and
Richard William Kerslake

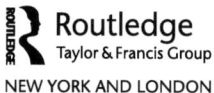
Routledge
Taylor & Francis Group

NEW YORK AND LONDON

First published 2024
by Routledge
605 Third Avenue, New York, NY 10158

and by Routledge
4 Park Square, Milton Park, Abingdon, Oxon, OX14 4RN

Routledge is an imprint of the Taylor & Francis Group, an informa business

Library of Congress Cataloging-in-Publication Data
Names: Bhaskaran, Arun, author. | Casper-Blake, Elijah, author. | Kerslake, Richard William, author.
Title: Revision guide for MRCPsych paper B / Arun Bhaskaran, Elijah Casper-Blake, Richard William Kerslake.
Description: New York, NY : Routledge, 2024. | Includes bibliographical references and index.
Identifiers: LCCN 2023025794 (print) | LCCN 2023025795 (ebook) | ISBN 9781032452548 (hardback) | ISBN 9781032452418 (paperback) | ISBN 9781003376163 (ebook)
Subjects: MESH: Psychiatry | Mental Disorders | Psychotherapy | Examination Questions
Classification: LCC RC480.5 (print) | LCC RC480.5 (ebook) | NLM WM 18.2 | DDC 616.89/14—dc23/eng/20230828
LC record available at https://lccn.loc.gov/2023025794
LC ebook record available at https://lccn.loc.gov/2023025795

ISBN: 978-1-032-45254-8 (hbk)
ISBN: 978-1-032-45241-8 (pbk)
ISBN: 978-1-003-37616-3 (ebk)

DOI: 10.4324/9781003376163

Typeset in Times New Roman
by Apex CoVantage, LLC

Contents

Acknowledgements

This book would not have been possible without the love and support of some very special people in our lives.

Arun would like to thank his fiancé, Matthew. His ambition and passion never cease to amaze and were major driving forces in completing this journey. Arun would also like to thank his siblings Aravin, Qasim and Joanne, who have stuck by his side through thick and thin, ups and downs and light and dark – writing this book being no exception.

Elijah would like to thank his friends and family for their uplifting words and tireless encouragement throughout this process. He would like to say a special thanks to his partner Danny for their faith and cheer. Words cannot express his gratitude.

Richard would like to give thanks to his parents and family for their unwavering support, his wife Taryn for her endless encouragement, and his children for their boundless inspiration.

Preface

This text was produced following the completion of our MRCPsych examinations. We feel that there are limited written texts currently available for students sitting the MRCPsych exams, and when we were revising, we struggled to find resources that matched the Royal College of Psychiatrists' syllabus. We often had to rely purely on online question banks or refer to multiple different sources to find information. We understand the challenges of juggling exam revision with work and life, and we want to help candidates revise smarter, not harder. We have created this book with those sitting their exams in mind. We wanted to create a resource to aid students in exam revision with relevant material in an easily accessible and readable format. We hope you find it a useful addition to your exam toolkit.

We wish you every success in your upcoming exam.

Arun, Elijah and Richard

1 Introduction and overview of the MRCPsych Paper B examination

Arun Arujun Bhaskaran

Greetings, peer and thank you for purchasing this revision guide!

This book is primarily aimed at doctors-in-training preparing for the Paper B component of their Member of the Royal College of Psychiatrists (MRCPsych) examinations. However, it can be good reference text for anyone working in a mental health setting or with patients suffering from mental health problems. Anyone with an interest in psychiatry and mental health might also find it a valuable addition to their bookcase.

About the MRCPsych examinations

The Royal College of Psychiatrists was established in 1971 with the objective of securing the best outcomes for patients with mental illness. One of its aims was to outline the knowledge and skills necessary for doctors wishing to specialise in psychiatry and treat such patients. The MRCPsych examinations assess this set of knowledge and skills and can be taken by any doctor in the UK, the European Union, or beyond. Refer to the MRCPsych Eligibility Criteria and Regulations on their website for further information[1].

The Paper B exam

The MRCPsych exams have seen a significant overhaul over recent years and currently consist of **2 written papers** (A and B) and the **CASC** (Clinical Assessment of Skills and Competencies). This revision guide focuses on Paper B, which can be sat by **any doctor in an approved training programme**. The Royal College recommends *12 months of experience in psychiatry* before sitting Paper B.

Paper B covers **critical review** and **clinical topics in psychiatry**. Each subsequent chapter in this book covers the sections outlined in the Paper B syllabus and offers a readable, comprehensive, and succinct set of revision notes that readers can use alongside other exam resources and question banks for self-testing in the lead-up to their exams. We understand the challenges of

DOI: 10.4324/9781003376163-1

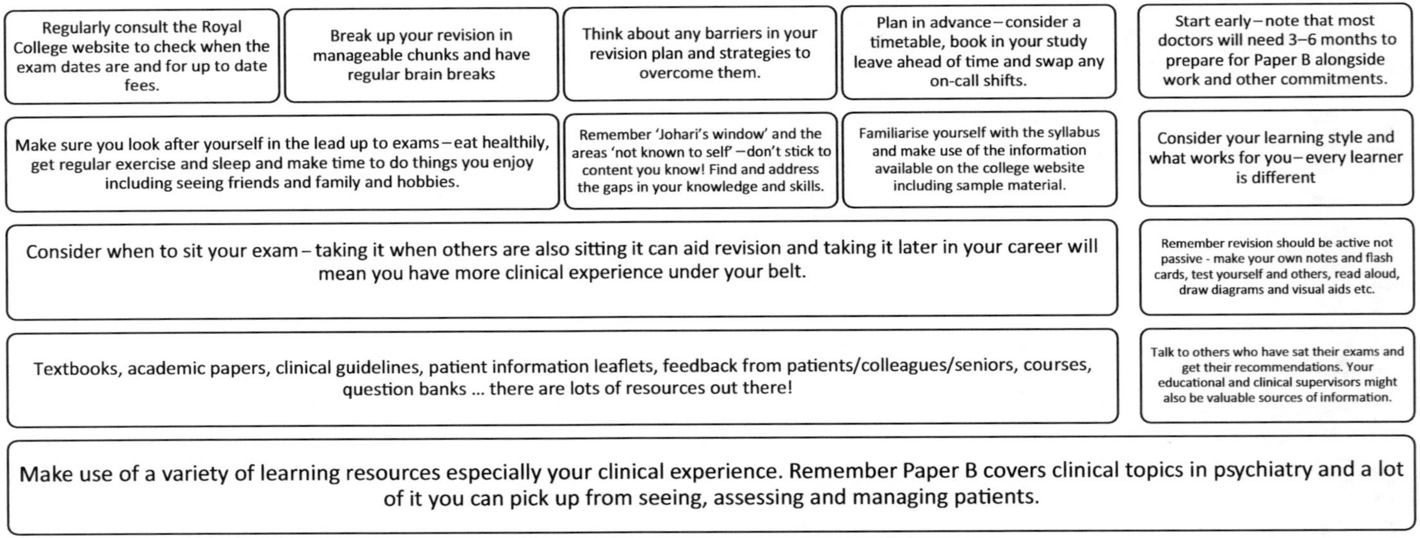

Start early—note that most doctors will need 3–6 months to prepare for Paper B alongside work and other commitments.

Consider your learning style and what works for you—every learner is different

Remember revision should be active not passive – make your own notes and flash cards, test yourself and others, read aloud, draw diagrams and visual aids etc.

Talk to others who have sat their exams and get their recommendations. Your educational and clinical supervisors might also be valuable sources of information.

Plan in advance—consider a timetable, book in your study leave ahead of time and swap any on-call shifts.

Familiarise yourself with the syllabus and make use of the information available on the college website including sample material.

Think about any barriers in your revision plan and strategies to overcome them.

Remember 'Johari's window' and the areas 'not known to self' – don't stick to content you know! Find and address the gaps in your knowledge and skills.

Consider when to sit your exam – taking it when others are also sitting it can aid revision and taking it later in your career will mean you have more clinical experience under your belt.

Regularly consult the Royal College website to check when the exam dates are and for up to date fees.

Break up your revision in manageable chunks and have regular brain breaks

Make sure you look after yourself in the lead up to exams – eat healthily, get regular exercise and sleep and make time to do things you enjoy including seeing friends and family and hobbies.

Textbooks, academic papers, clinical guidelines, patient information leaflets, feedback from patients/colleagues/seniors, courses, question banks … there are lots of resources out there!

Make use of a variety of learning resources especially your clinical experience. Remember Paper B covers clinical topics in psychiatry and a lot of it you can pick up from seeing, assessing and managing patients.

Figure 1.1 Tips and advice from fellow psychiatrists

juggling exam revision with working and other aspects of daily life, and we want to help readers work smarter not harder.

Following the COVID-19 pandemic and the College's efforts to avoid disruptions to the exams, the Paper B exam is digitalised and currently **taken online**.

At the time of writing, Paper B is a **3-hour examination** consisting of **150** multiple choice (**MCQ**) and extended matching questions (**EMQ**).

The rough stratification of questions outlined by the Royal College is as follows:

Table 1.1 Breakdown of Paper B exam

Organisation and delivery of psychiatric services, psychotherapy, forensic psychiatry and psychiatry of learning disability	5.5% each
Old age psychiatry and child and adolescent psychiatry	9% each
Substance misuse and addictions	6.5%
General adult psychiatry	20%
Critical review	33.5%

Advice from us for preparing for Paper B

> *Finally, we wish you the best of luck in your exams and hope this book is a helpful tool in creating your path to success*

> *– Arun, Elijah and Richard*

Reference

1. Preparing for Exams. *Royal College of Psychiatrists*. rcpsych.ac.uk. Accessed 03/01/2023

2 Organisation and delivery of psychiatric services

Elijah Casper-Blake

Preventative strategies in mental health

Risk factors for mental illness[1,30]

Public mental health is an expanding field in psychiatry.

Risk factors for mental illness are wide-ranging and can relate to a variety of factors:

- Genetics – Most conditions are thought to have a genetic aspect to them.

    - Bipolar affective disorder has an 85% heritability and major depression disorder has a 37% heritability.
    - Some conditions may be directly linked to chromosomal abnormalities, e.g., Down syndrome.

- Early life and family environment

    - Pregnancy – Maternal wellbeing during pregnancy, infections, substance misuse and pregnancy-related complications.
    - Parental mental health – Parental mental illness increases the risks of mental illness in offspring.
    - Poor family relationships and attachment.
    - Abuse – All types of abuse increase the risk of adult mental health problems. Childhood sexual abuse has been found to increase the risk of depression (odds ratio (OR) 2.04), psychosis (OR 2.38) and bipolar affective disorder (OR 2.58).
    - Childhood adversity – Childhood difficulties could account for 30% of adult mental health problems.
    - Education – Poor education is linked to a higher risk of mental disorders.

- Individual factors

    - Individual personality factors – high neuroticism, low extraversion and low conscientiousness – can increase risk of burnout, social isolation and use of maladaptive coping strategies.

DOI: 10.4324/9781003376163-2

- Physical illness – Depression rates increase 2-fold in individuals with common medical problems and 7-fold in individuals with more than 1 physical health condition.
- Stressful life events.
- (Un)employment – Employment can provide both a source of stress and source of support. However, unemployment confers an increased risk of depression and suicide.
- Substance misuse
- Finances – A source of stress for most, there are higher rates of mental illness in those with lower incomes, this is true for both adults and children in the household.
- Sleep – Insomnia increases the risk of mental illness.

- Societal and socioeconomic factors

  - Inequality – Children from disadvantaged backgrounds are 2–3x more likely to develop mental illness.
  - Living environment – Quality and safety of an individuals' living environment and housing and access to green space have been shown in research to have an impact on mental health.
  - Crime – Crime can be a direct precipitant for illness such as post-traumatic stress disorder (PTSD).
  - Social isolation – Increasing loneliness in society can impact on social support networks, impairing resilience and helpful coping strategies and perpetuate existing mental health difficulties.
  - Impact of the environment – Air pollution has been linked to an increased risk of psychosis and mental disorders; environmental catastrophes and climate change can be direct stressors.

Public health intervention[1,31]

Intervention strategies in public mental health can be classified by who they target on an individual or population level along with the stage of a condition that they target.

Condition:

- **Primary prevention** – Intervention aimed to prevent a condition from arising – e.g., antenatal vitamins, health education/promotion such as drug and alcohol prevention strategies.
- **Secondary prevention** – Intervention for those in at-risk or asymptomatic populations – e.g., early intervention in psychosis, screening programmes.
- **Tertiary prevention** – Prevention of relapse or further problems for those who have a diagnosed condition – e.g., Aspirin to manage stroke/myocardial infarction (MI) risk, depot injections, smoking cessation.

Population:

- **Universal prevention** – An intervention that impacts the whole population to reduce risk of a condition – e.g., fortification of food products and tap water.
- **Selective prevention** – An intervention that targets a specific population – e.g., human immunodeficiency virus (HIV) screening in high-risk areas or populations.

Psychiatric services

Introduction[1,2,4,5]

- Around 1/4 of the adult population is affected by mental disorders each year
- The Adult Psychiatric Morbidity Survey of 2014 indicated that:
  - 1 in 6 adults aged 16 and over had experienced a common mental health difficulty in the past week.
  - Only 46.4% of individuals with common mental health disorders had discussed them with their general practitioner (GP) in the last year.
  - 20.6% of individuals with common mental disorders accessed mental health services, including community mental health services, therapy and third-sector services.
  - Only 4.9% of individuals with a common mental disorder saw a psychiatrist.
  - Rates for accessing treatment varied depending on illness, with 82.4% of individuals with psychosis having accessed treatment within the last year.
  - This suggests that whilst many individuals do access, treatment there are many members of the community who may have unmet needs and indeed many individuals with mental illness who do not end up in a psychiatrist clinic.

Mental health support and services

- Individuals in the community may seek support from a variety of services.
- Around 3 in 4 individuals with mental health problems will be managed by their GP without being referred to secondary mental health services.

Charitable and third-sector organisations

- Many voluntary and community organisations provide invaluable support for individuals with mental health difficulties.
- These organisations often offer a diverse range of support from mental health specific groups such as Mind to more activity- or employment-focused organisations.

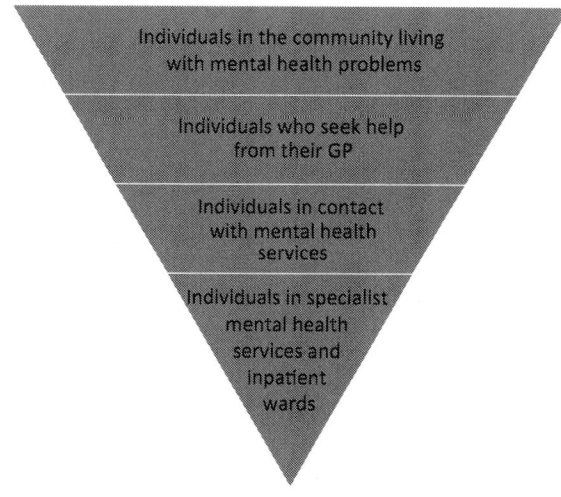

Figure 2.1 Distribution of individuals with mental health problems

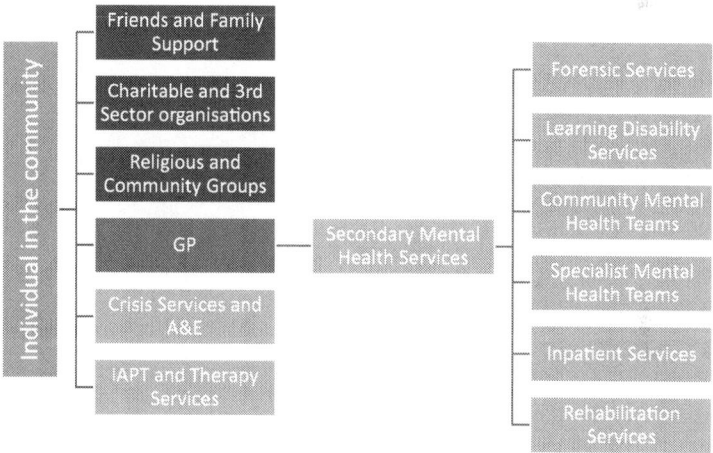

Figure 2.2 Mental health support in the community

- These organisations can provide education and support in an accessible form.
- Individuals may find it easier to relate to an organisation that sits outside of the medical sphere.

Secondary mental health services[4,5]

Mental health services in the community as well as inpatient services tend to be divided between the following groups:

- Child and adolescent mental health services – For individuals under the age of 18.

- Older adult services – These services have different criteria dependent on the team; however, they are set up to support older adults (generally aged either 65+ or 70+), especially those with dementia or frailty.
- Forensic services – These work closely with the Ministry of Justice for individuals with a forensic history. Please see Chapter 8 of this book for further details.
- Learning disability services – These services are set up specifically for individuals with a diagnosed or suspected learning disability; they have different criteria depending on the team.
- General adult services – For individuals aged 18+ who do not otherwise fit the criteria for the aforementioned services.

The multidisciplinary team (MDT)

Psychiatric teams are generally comprised of a broad range of professionals to offer wholistic support to individuals.

The following is a list of professionals you might expect to see on an MDT:

- Psychiatrists.
- Psychiatric nurses.
- Social workers.
- Occupational therapists.
- Support workers.
- Psychologists and psychotherapists.
- Support workers.
- Peer workers – Individuals with lived experience of mental health problems.
- Administration team.

Care plan approach (CPA)[3]

- The CPA is a framework initially set out in 1991 to support individuals with complex mental health needs.
- Its aim was to introduce a person-centred recovery plan and provide a level of continuity of care.
- The CPA is being replaced by the common mental health framework.
- Key components of this are:

    - A comprehensive, wholistic care plan compiled with an individual and the professionals involved in their care.
    - Regular review of the care plan (usually every 6 months).
    - A care co-ordinator who is a regular point of contact within the team working with an individual.

In addition to members of the MDT, mental health services often work closely with hospital specialists such as paediatricians, geriatricians, neurologists and radiologists, as well as GPs.

Community mental health teams

Different areas within the country seem to have different layouts of their community services; however, most have a version of what is called a community mental health team. These teams tend to manage the majority of individuals who have been referred to mental health services.

- Community mental health teams tend to support individuals with severe mental illness whilst providing advice and support to primary care.
- Community mental health teams may offer assessment and diagnosis.
- Community mental health teams can provide advice and support around management to primary care and other services.
- Community mental health teams can provide longer-term care for individuals who require ongoing support.
- Individuals may be seen solely by a psychiatrist, whilst individuals with more complex or specialist needs may be supported by other team members.
- Individuals with higher support needs may be supported with by care co-ordinators.

Teams for specialist conditions

- Some conditions or groups are managed by specialist teams to provide specialist diagnosis or management of a condition.
- Examples include:
  - Adult ADHD and autism.
  - Memory clinics – dementia.
  - Personality disorder services.
  - Eating disorder teams.

Early intervention in psychosis (EIP) teams[1,6]

The National Institute for Health and Care Excellence (NICE) guidelines recommend that early intervention services be made available to all individuals who are experiencing a first episode of psychosis and that these services be made available for up to 3 years for individuals who require their support.

Their goal is to provide rapid access to diagnosis and treatment alongside a range of additional services including psychology, education and occupational support, alongside social interventions.

Mental Health National Service Framework

- This was a framework set out in 1999 to establish priorities within of mental health care in the UK.
- It set out 5 key areas to set national standards on:
  - Mental health promotion.
  - Primary care and access to services.
  - Effective services for people with severe mental illness.
  - Caring about caregivers.
  - Preventing suicide.
- It initially had a broad scope, which had to be narrowed, but was key to the promotion of:
  - Crisis teams.
  - Assertive outreach teams.
  - Early intervention teams.

EIP teams are supported by data suggesting that:

- Individuals with a longer duration of untreated psychosis have a worse outcome both symptomatically and in terms of return to social functioning.
- Individuals under EIP services are less likely to be admitted to hospital and may have a reduced burden of psychotic symptoms.
- Individuals under EIP services are 116% more likely to be employed and 52% more likely to be in mainstream housing compared to those who are not receiving input.
- Individuals under EIP are no less likely to relapse, but may have a better long-term outcome.

Assertive outreach teams[4,7]

Assertive outreach teams were part of the Mental Health National Service Framework, and whilst they remain in some areas, their services have been greatly reduced.

The approach is based around trying to proactively engage individuals who have complex mental health needs.

They were designed to support individuals who had:

- A history of violence or offence.
- Significant risk of self-harm or self-neglect.
- Treatment resistance.
- Dual diagnosis – Substance misuse and mental health illness.

Key components of the programme of assertive community treatment approach

- Persistent and proactive approaches to engagement.
- Comprehensive assessments of patients' needs and goals.
- Teamworking and care co-ordination.
- Daily reviews of the caseload within the team.
- 7-day access to the team, ability to respond rapidly and crisis intervention.
- Empowering independence and supporting building of social networks.
- Supporting families and caregivers.
- Medication support and administration if required.
- Treating comorbidities.
- Physical health monitoring.
- Relapse prevention.

- A history of detainment under the mental health act within the last 2 years.
- A history of homelessness or unstable housing situations.

Assertive outreach teams are an intensive engagement and apply a wholistic approach to supporting an individual.

- Caseloads are typically 1 professional to 10 service users.
- They are a costly intervention due to this significant involvement, but were brought in due to research that suggests that they result in better outcomes and fewer hospitalisations.

Crisis and home treatment teams

- Crisis services are designed to support people in a crisis and to help provide rapid treatment and risk containment.
- Crisis services can be accessed directly by members of the public usually by 24/7 phone lines, alongside specific referrals by mental health professionals.
- Crisis services can provide one-off support, but they also tend to offer a short period of regular (often daily) interventions to support an individual.
- Crisis teams are intended to support those who might otherwise require a hospital admission to be managed in the community.
- They often play a role in facilitating hospital admission in individuals who require this.

Recovery and rehabilitation teams[5,8,9]

Rehabilitation services are set up to help individuals recover from episodes of severe mental illness (generally psychotic illnesses) that have a significant impact on day-to-day functioning.

NICE recommends referral to rehabilitation services for individuals who have "complex psychosis" and are identified as having treatment-resistant symptoms and functional impairment. Such services are particularly recommended for those who have had multiple admissions to hospital as well as those with difficulties living in the community.

The recovery-orientated approach

Recovery means different things to different people, and the recovery orientated approach is based around helping someone achieve their individual goals and lead a meaningful life despite mental illness. This is a holistic approach focusing not simply on the resolution of the symptoms of mental illness but including areas such as housing, building social structures, wellbeing and education.

Key principles include:

- Optimism and hope for recovery
- Empowering individuals to achieve their own goals
- Focus on the individual as opposed to the mental illness
- Promoting independence
- Understanding that recovery is not a straight path and may be different for each individual

---

Rehabilitation services often include a mixture of both inpatient settings and outpatient community teams or day hospitals.

The focus of rehabilitation services is to help individuals to regain their confidence and gain skills whilst feeling empowered. They are generally led by a recovery-orientated approach.

Rehabilitation services generally offer a variety of interventions including:

- Medication – Support around finding the right medication regimen, alongside support around medication engagement.
- Psychological therapies.
- Activities – Social activities such as gardening and crafts.
- Support around physical health and substance misuse.
- Living skills training – Money management, cooking and cleaning, amongst others.

- Education and occupational support.
- Housing and accommodation.

Psychological services

- People in different regions may have varying access to psychological therapies.
- NHS talking therapies (formerly Improving Access to Psychological Therapies (IAPT)) is an intervention to provide improved access to evidence-based talking therapies with trained professionals. It provides stepped care for individuals with common mental disorders and is generally available by self-referral. Typical interventions include cognitive behavioural therapy (CBT) and behavioural activation[10].
- Individual trusts may have their own dedicated psychotherapy teams, and the type of therapy may vary by trust.
- Individual teams such as community mental health, rehabilitation and EIP teams often have in-house psychologists to provide specialist input.

Inpatient wards[37]

- Each NHS trust has its own inpatient ward for care of individuals who need the additional support of a ward environment.
- Inpatient wards are often divided between patient groups, e.g., separate wards for older adults, working-age adults.
- In 2018/2019, the number of inpatient mental health beds in England was 18,400.
- There has been a significant decrease in the number of beds over time. This in part is due to the trend towards managing more individuals at home where possible with services such as home treatment teams.

Mental health, individual rights and medicolegal concerns

Mental Capacity Act 2005[32]

The mental capacity act governs an individual's ability to make decisions on their own behalf.

- All individuals are assumed to have capacity unless otherwise proven.
- Every attempt must be made to ensure an individual is able to understand a decision, e.g., using different methods of communication.
- Individuals are entitled to make unwise decisions.
- Any intervention undertaken with those who lack capacity must be in their best interest and the least restrictive option.

Capacity assessment

The capacity assessment is a 2-step process:

1) Does an individual have an "impairment of, or a disturbance in the functioning of, the mind or brain" that means they are unable to make a decision at that time?
2) An individual is classed as being unable to make a decision if they cannot do any of the following:

  - Understand the information relevant to the decision.
  - Retain the information.
  - Use the relevant information to weigh up their decision.
  - Communicate (in any form) their decision.

Deprivation of liberties safeguards (DOLS)[33]

What is a deprivation of liberty?

- If an individual is restricted or not free to leave or is under continuous supervision or control but lacks capacity to consent to this, then this amounts to a **Deprivation of Liberties**.
- This restriction can be physical, environmental or in the form of medical restraint.
- An example would be someone living with dementia in a care home who is not free to leave.

DOLS are specific protections put in place for individuals whose liberty has been restricted.

- Once established, individuals under DOLS must have an assessment by 2 professionals independent from their care team who must review the individual's capacity and the appropriateness of this measure. These 2 individuals are:

  - **Best interest assessor** (trained allied professional).
  - **Trained mental health doctor**.

- There must be **regular reviews** of an individual's care.
- Efforts should be sought to gain the **input of friends, relatives** or an independent mental capacity advocate (**IMCA**).
- All decisions made should be in line with the principles set out in the mental capacity act – They should be made in the individual's best interest, with previously expressed views considered, and in the least restrictive way possible.
- Individuals have the right to appeal decisions made.

DOLS are in the process of being **replaced** by **liberty protection safeguards**.

Advanced decisions[34]

Lasting power of attorney (LPA):

- Allows others to make a decision on the individual's behalf.
- 2 types – Health and welfare (daily care needs, health decisions, placement in care homes) versus property and financial affairs.
- Individual must have capacity when they nominate someone for their LPA.
- All decisions must be made in an individual's best interest, respecting their previous wishes or instructions and their human rights.

Human rights act 1998[35]

- The human rights act sets out fundamental human rights that are acknowledged by the state. Articles 2–12 and 14 set out the rights that all citizens are entitled to.
- Note that Article 1 and 13 are not present as they relate to the application of these fundamental rights.

There are a number of ways in which psychiatrists may interact with the Human Rights Act

- **Article 2 – The right to life.**

  - Individuals have a right to their own life and for this not to be endangered by others. Authorities have a requirement to safeguard life.
  - Authorities must investigate suspicious deaths.
  - Psychiatrists may need to make decisions around risks posed to others.

- **Article 3 – Freedom from torture and inhumane and degrading treatment.**

  - Organisations are required to be involved in safeguarding processes.
  - There are legal frameworks guiding how individuals can be treated regarding the use of restraint and seclusion.

- **Article 4 – Freedom from slavery and forced labour.**

  - Organisations are required to be involved in safeguarding processes.

- **Article 5 – Right to liberty and security.**

  - Individuals have the right to their own freedom unless there are adequate reasons, e.g., in the case of a crime, spread of infectious disease or mental illness.
  - Psychiatrists may play a role in involuntary detention and restriction of individual's liberties under the mental health act and mental capacity act/DOLS framework.

- **Article 6 – Right to a fair trial.**

  - Individuals detained under the mental health act have the ability to appeal their detention and be heard at a mental health act or hospital tribunal.

- **Article 7 – No punishment without law.**

  - An act must be a crime at the time it was committed to be found guilty of breaking the law and any punishment given must be in line with the law of that time.

- **Article 8 – Respect for your private and family life, home and correspondence.**

  - Right of an individual to privacy whilst under services or in hospital.
  - Right to make decisions around treatment and care.
  - Right of individuals supported by care services to a private life.

- **Article 9 – Freedom of thought, belief and religion.**

  - Respect for and understanding of aspects of cultural psychiatry.
  - Provision or access to religious practice whilst someone is detained.

- **Article 10 – Freedom of expression.**

  - Individuals are encouraged to make shared decisions around their care.
  - Individuals detained in a hospital environment may have limited access to methods of communication.

- **Article 11 – Freedom of assembly and association.**

  - The freedom of individuals to assemble and join in groups such as trade unions or political parties.

- **Article 12 – Right to marry and start a family.**

  - The rights of individuals supported by care services to a family.

- **Article 14 – Protection from discrimination in respect of these rights and freedoms.**

  - Psychiatrists should be aware of institutional discrimination within the mental health system.

Tarasoff case

- A 1974 case from California, USA.
- The case centres around the murder of Tatiana Tarasoff.

- Ms Tarasoff's murderer had allegedly disclosed his intentions to kill her 2 months prior to his psychologist.
- The court ruled that although Ms Tarasoff was not under the care of the psychologist, that they had a duty and legal obligation to warn her of this significant danger.
- This case is often cited when discussing the **"duty to warn."**

Confidentiality[11–13]

All individuals are entitled to their personal information to be kept in a safe manner and to expect that it remains confidential.

In the doctor–patient relationship, this is vital to enable individuals to feel they are able to disclose important and often personal information to aid in diagnosis and management.

Doctors have both a **legal** and an **ethical duty to keep this confidentiality**.

There are, however, some cases where professionals can or are compelled to share this information:

- Where individuals have capacity and consent to their data being shared.
- Where individuals lack capacity to consent to their information being shared but it is deemed to be in their best interest.
- In public health interests – e.g., certain notifiable diseases.
- Safeguarding – Where others are risk of harm or abuse.
- Female genital mutilation – If this is identified in children under as 18.
- Regulatory bodies, the Driving and Vehicle Licensing Agency (DVLA), by direction of the secretary of state and for counter fraud purposes.
- Court order.
- To prevent serious crime or threats towards and individual or national security.

The British Medical Association (BMA) and General Medical Council (GMC) both offer guides to capacity and the disclosure of information.

Any disclosure of information against an individual's consent should be discussed with senior members of the team and advice can be sought from the trust **Caldicot Guardian**.

Driving and mental disorders[36]

The following chart is taken from the first book in this series, "Revision Guide for MRCPsych Paper A."

Mild to moderate anxiety and depression	May drive, and the DVLA does not need to be notified as long as there are no significant deficits in cognition or concentration, or risk for agitation or suicidal thoughts.
Severe anxiety and depression	Must not drive and must notify the DVLA.
Acute psychotic disorder	Must not drive during acute illness and must notify the DVLA.
Mania	Must not drive and must notify the DVLA during acute illness but can drive after a manic episode if certain conditions are met.
Schizophrenia	Must not drive and must notify the DVLA during acute illness but can drive after a psychotic episode if certain conditions are met.
Mild cognitive impairment	May drive and the DVLA does not need to be notified.
Dementia	Must notify the DVLA. There is acknowledgement that dementia can present in different ways with alternative rates of progression, and the decision regarding licensing is usually based on medical reports with review as necessary.
Mild learning disability	Must notify the DVLA. Licensing will be granted providing there are no other significant relevant problems.
Severe learning disability	Must NOT drive and must notify the DVLA.

Abuse of adults[14-18]

Abuse is the **maltreatment** or **exploitation** of a person, and can include **intentional harm** or the **failure** to **prevent** it.

All professionals working in the health and social care section have a duty to safeguard service users and to report concerns around risks of abuse.

Safeguarding refers to the actions taken to protect an individual from abuse or harm as well as those that are vulnerable and at risk of this.

Individual organisations will have their own safeguarding policies alongside safeguarding leads which can provide support and advice in cases where abuse is suspected.

The **Care Act of 2014** sets out key principles around safeguarding:

- **Empowerment** of an individual regarding their care.
- **Protection** of victims of abuse.
- **Prevention** of harm where abuse is suspected or the individual is at risk.
- **Proportionality** dependent on the individual and situation.
- **Partnership** with appropriate organisations.
- **Accountability** of organisations and understanding the roles they play.

Under the Care Act, local authorities have a duty to investigate any cases where an individual who has care needs is felt to be at risk of or is experiencing abuse and neglect. They are required to consider whether action needs to be taken as a result. This is called a **Section 42 enquiry.**

Where does abuse take place?

2021–2022 figures for the location of Section 42 enquiries show:

- 48% took place in the home – the most common area.
- 22.7% took place in residential homes.
- 9.5% took place in nursing homes.
- 4.1% took place in the community.
- 3.4% took place in acute medical hospitals.
- 3.2% took place in mental health hospitals.
- 6% took place in other areas.

Categories of abuse

- Physical abuse – Including physical acts of aggression, physical restraint, misuse of medications.
- Emotional/psychological abuse – intimidation and threats, coercive or controlling behaviours, humiliation, withdrawal from support or social groups.
- Domestic abuse – This includes different forms of abuse specifically directed towards individuals who have been or are still in a relationship or other family members.
- Sexual abuse – Rape, inappropriate sexual contact, abuse of positions of trust, sexual coercion, exposure to sexual material without an individual's consent.
- Financial abuse – Theft or misuse of money, pressuring an individual around their finances, scamming.
- Neglect and acts of omission – Not giving an individual the basic needs that they require, e.g., food and care needs.
- Self-neglect – Not caring for one's own self.
- Discriminatory abuse – Abuse on the grounds of an individual's characteristics, e.g., race, sex, sexuality.
- Organisational/institutional – Practices or cultures within an organisation that result in neglect or abuse of another kind.
- Modern slavery – Human trafficking and forced labour.

Specific treatments in mental health

Electroconvulsive therapy (ECT)[19,23]

Origins

- Seizure therapy has its origins in the 1930's.
- ECT was first introduced by **Ugo Cerletti** and **Lucio Bini**.

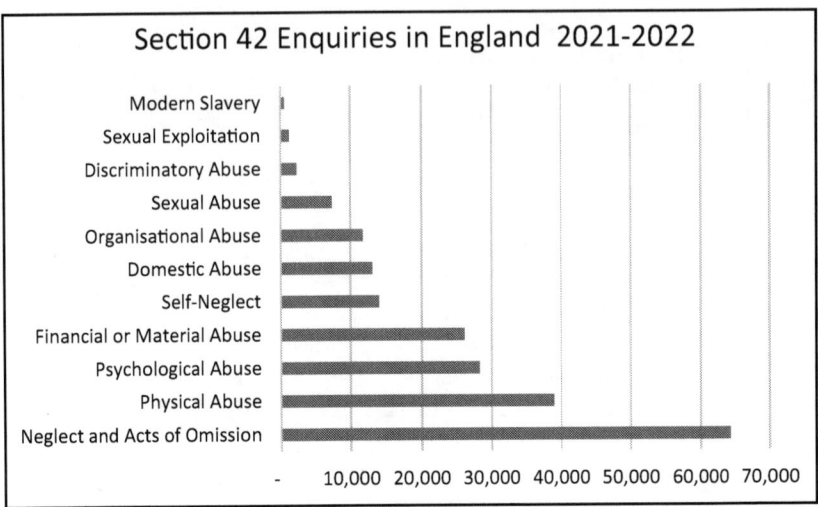

Figure 2.3 Distribution and number of Section 42 enquiries that were undertaken in England between 2021 and 2022

- Prior to this, however, chemicals had been used to induce seizures, as introduced by **Ladislas von Meduna**.

Mechanism of action

The mechanism of action of ECT is not fully understood, but some different hypotheses have been put forward:

- Changes in cerebral blood flow and blood brain barrier permeability.
- Changes in neurochemical pathways including the release of various neurochemicals and expression of neuroreceptors.
- Release of growth factors which can promote neuroplasticity in connectivity.

How is an ECT clinic run[20]

- ECT will generally take place in a dedicated clinic within a hospital.
- A framework for standards of care within ECT clinics is set out by the ECT Accreditation Service (ECTAS) covering all aspects of the procedure.
- Clinics staff will include:
  - Psychiatrist.
  - Anaesthetist.
  - Operating department practitioner (ODP).
  - Nursing staff and recovery staff.

- A course of ECT typically lasts for around **6–12 sessions** which are given **twice a week**.
- Some individuals may continue to have regular sessions which are classed as **maintenance ECT**.

Prior to undergoing ECT

- A full assessment of an individual's mental health and the indication for ECT should be performed.
- Assessment of capacity to consent to the procedure or relevant assessment under the mental health act should take place (see below).
- Physical health assessment

  - Anaesthetic review.
  - Blood tests.
  - Electrocardiogram.
  - Chest X-ray.

The procedure

- Individuals should not eat or drink for 6 hours prior to the procedure.
- Benzodiazepine drugs and lithium are typically withheld prior to the procedure.
- Individuals will arrive at the ECT clinic and have an initial assessment with the psychiatrist including:

  - Review of their mental health.
  - Review of their capacity to consent.
  - Cognitive assessment.
  - Discussion of progress of the treatment, including any side effects and whether the treatment has been helpful.
  - Discussion of current physical health problems.

- The procedure will take place in a clinic room and typically last around **1 hour**.
- Vital signs alongside electroencephalogram readouts will be continuously monitored through the procedure.
- An anaesthetist will administer an anaesthetic and muscle relaxant, providing oxygen if required.
- Two electrodes can be placed either **bilaterally** or **unilaterally.**
- An electrical pulse is administered to provoke a seizure.
- The **seizure** typically **lasts around 40 seconds**.
- Following this, individuals are supported in a recovery area with close monitoring before leaving the clinic.

Capacity and consent[21]

- ECT is covered under section 58A of the mental health act.
- ECT is appropriate for individuals with the capacity to make relevant decisions.

  - ECT can be given with patient consent, but individuals **under the age of 18 must be assessed by a second opinion appointed doctor (SOAD).**
  - If they do not consent to the procedure, it cannot take place.

- Individuals who lack capacity to make decisions around ECT:

  - Must be assessed by a SOAD to confirm that they lack capacity.
  - The SOAD must also check that no legal arrangement such as advanced decisions, court orders or nominated deputies object to the treatment.

Indications[22,24]

ECT is an effective treatment used to achieve rapid improvement for individuals with severe symptoms which have not responded to other treatments or in cases which are life threatening.

NICE guidance recommends ECT in the following conditions:

- **Prolonged mania** not responding to medication.
- **Catatonia**
- **Depression**

  - When a rapid response is required due to individual risks.
  - When other treatments have not been successful.
  - Where a service user requests this because it has been helpful in the past.

- **Schizophrenia**

  - ECT **is not recommended** for general use in individuals with schizophrenia who do not meet the aforementioned criteria.

Contraindications

- There are **no absolute contraindications** to ECT.

Relative contraindications

- Current respiratory illness.
- Vascular aneurysms.
- Recent intracranial haemorrhage or infraction.

- Arrythmia.
- Recent myocardial infarction.
- Retinal detachment.

Side effects[20,22]

- Headache.
- Nausea.
- Muscle pains and aches.
- Peripheral nerve palsy.
- Status epilepticus.
- Mortality – The mortality rate is no more than that of other anaesthetic procedures and is said to be around 1/50,000–1/100,000.

ECT and memory

- The extent to which ECT impacts memory, particularly in the longer term, is a topic of debate.
- Memory loss of the immediate events surrounding an ECT treatment is common (40%).
- Some individuals may report more prolonged difficulties with their memories, which generally resolve.
- Severe depression and other mental health conditions will also have an impact on memory.
- Some individuals do report longer-term problems with their memory; however, this is thought to be a small number.
- ECT **does not increase the risk of dementia** in the long term.

Outcomes

- ECT, by the nature of its indication, is generally only used in individuals with severe symptoms of mental health conditions.
- In a survey, 68% of people said they were much improved or very much improved following treatment with ECT.

Psychosurgery[19,25,26]

Introduction

- Psychosurgery began in 1936 and was pioneered by **Egas Moniz (frontal leucotomy)**.
- Psychosurgery continues to be used in a small number of patients.
- Psychosurgery is performed in specialist centres (The UK has centres in London and Dundee).

- Modern psychosurgery involves the precise ablation of specific parts of the brain guided by magnetic resonance imaging or computerised tomography.

Indications

- Psychosurgery is typically reserved for individuals who have not responded to all other alternatives.
- The Royal College of Psychiatrists states that it can be helpful in "carefully selected patients" with:

  - **Obsessive-compulsive disorder (OCD).**
  - **Depression.**
  - There is limited evidence for its use in other conditions.

Procedures

The most common procedures offered are:

- **Anterior cingulotomy** – This involves bilateral incisions to affect the cingulate gyrus.
- **Anterior capsulotomy** – This involves bilateral incisions to affect the anterior limb of the internal capsule.

Capacity and consent[21]

- Psychosurgery is covered under **Section 57** of the mental health act.
- Psychosurgery **cannot** be performed on those who **do not consent** to it.
- **Capacity** to consent to treatment **must be assessed** by a **SOAD** and **2 independent clinicians** who are not doctors.

Side effects and complications

- Headache.
- Confusion.
- Loss of memory for the immediate post-operative period.
- Loss of control of the bladder (usually short-term).
- Weight gain.
- Brain haemorrhage.
- Infection.
- Epileptic seizures.
- It is **not** thought to cause **changes in personality** or **cognition**.

Outcomes

- 63% of individuals with depression showed marked improvement.

- 58% of individuals with OCD showed marked improvement.

Repetitive transcranial magnetic stimulation (rTMS)[19,27,28]

Overview

- rTMS is a relatively new, non-invasive technique in psychiatry.
- rTMS makes use of an electromagnetic coil that is placed on the scalp and is induced to create an electromagnetic field.
- **Repetitive** pulses stimulate the electromagnetic coil and have an impact on neuronal activity.
- Individuals are awake and alert whilst the procedure takes place.
- Treatment is given **5 days a week** for a period of around **2–6 weeks**.

Indications

- **Depression** – NICE Guidance suggests that there is evidence for its use in the short term.
- There is less evidence for other conditions, although there is interest in its use in conditions such as OCD and schizophrenia.

Contraindications

- Cochlear implants.
- Cardiac pacemakers.
- Presence of metal in the patient's head.
- Epilepsy.

Side effects

- Headache.
- Scalp pain.
- Muscle twitching (during procedure).
- Tinnitus and hearing problems.
- Hypomania.
- Seizures.

Other techniques of neuromodulation

Vagus nerve stimulation[25,29]

OVERVIEW

- The use of vagal nerve stimulators in psychiatry comes from observations of their use in individuals with epilepsy.

- The stimulation device can be either **transcutaneous** or **implanted**.
- These devices tend to stimulate the vagus nerve in the neck.
- Their use has been proposed in individuals with **depression**.
- There is limited evidence for their use at this time, and their routine use outside of research is not recommended.

Deep brain stimulation

- Deep brain stimulation has been used in the treatment of Parkinson's disease.
- Its use has also been suggested in **OCD** and **depression**.
- The most common technique suggested is the direct stimulation of nuclei by implanted electrodes in the **internal capsule** and **cingulate cortex**.
- At this time, there is not enough evidence for routine use outside of research.

References

1. Public mental health: Evidence, practice and commissioning. *Royal College of Psychiatrists*, May 2019, www.rsph.org.uk/static/uploaded/b215d040-2753-410e-a39eb30ad3c8b708.pdf
2. Adult psychiatric morbidity survey: Survey of mental health and wellbeing, England, 2014, 29 September 2016, https://digital.nhs.uk/data-and-information/publications/statistical/adult-psychiatric-morbidity-survey/adult-psychiatric-morbidity-survey-survey-of-mental-health-and-wellbeing-england-2014
3. Care for people with mental health problems (Care Programme Approach), March 2021. *NHS Website*, www.nhs.uk/conditions/social-care-and-support-guide/help-from-social-services-and-charities/care-for-people-with-mental-health-problems-care-programme-approach/
4. A national service framework for mental health. *UK Government*, September 1999, https://assets.publishing.service.gov.uk/government/uploads/system/uploads/attachment_data/file/198051/National_Service_Framework_for_Mental_Health.pdf
5. Paul Harrison, Philip Cowen, Tom Burns, Mina Fazel. Chapter 26. Psychiatric services. In *Shorter oxford textbook of psychiatry*. 7th edition. Oxford University Press.
6. NICE Guidelines 178. Psychosis and schizophrenia in adults: Prevention and management, March 2014, www.nice.org.uk/guidance/cg178/chapter/Recommendations#preventing-psychosis-2
7. Department of Health. *Mental health implementation guide*. Department of Health, 2010.
8. NICE Guidelines 181. Rehabilitation for adults with complex psychosis, August 2020, www.nice.org.uk/guidance/ng181/chapter/Recommendations
9. Royal college of psychiatrists. *Mental Health Rehabilitation Services*, www.rcpsych.ac.uk/mental-health/treatments-and-wellbeing/mental-health-rehabilitation-services
10. NHS talking therapies. *NHS England*, www.england.nhs.uk/mental-health/adults/nhs-talking-therapies/
11. Tarasoff v. Regents of Univ. of Cal. – 13 Cal. 3d 177, 118 Cal. Rptr. 129, 529 P. 2d 553 (Cal. 1974), lexis nexis, www.lexisnexis.com/community/casebrief/p/casebrief-tarasoff-v-regents-of-univ-of-cal

12. BMA Confidentiality and health records toolkit, July 2021, www.bma.org.uk/media/4283/bma-confidentiality-and-health-records-toolkit-july-2021.pdf

13. Confidentiality good practice in handling patient information. *GMC*, www.gmc-uk.org/-/media/documents/gmc-guidance-for-doctors – confidentiality-good-practice-in-handling-patient-information–70080105.pdf

14. Care act 2014, legislation.gov.uk, www.legislation.gov.uk/ukpga/2014/23/contents/enacted

15. College safeguarding policy and procedures. *Royal College of Psychiatrists*, July 2022, www.rcpsych.ac.uk/docs/default-source/about-us/safeguarding/rcpsych-safeguarding-policy – hr-december–2020.pdf

16. SD8: Office of the Public Guardian safeguarding policy. *Office of the Guardian*, January 2023, www.gov.uk/government/publications/safeguarding-policy-protecting-vulnerable-adults/sd8-opgs-safeguarding-policy#opgs-role-in-safeguarding-adults-at-risk

17. Safeguarding adult. *NHS England*, www.england.nhs.uk/wp-content/uploads/2017/02/adult-pocket-guide.pdf

18. Safeguarding adults England 2021–2022. *NHS England*, August 2022, https://digital.nhs.uk/data-and-information/publications/statistical/safeguarding-adults/2021-22

19. Paul Harrison, Philip Cowen, Tom Burns, Mina Fazel. Chapter 25 drugs and other physical treatments. In Michael G. Gelder (eds.), *Shorter Oxford textbook of psychiatry*, 7th edition. Oxford University Press.

20. Electroconvulsive therapy. *Royal College of Psychiatrists*, www.rcpsych.ac.uk/mental-health/treatments-and-wellbeing/ect

21. The mental health act 1983: Code of practice. *Department of Health*, https://assets.publishing.service.gov.uk/government/uploads/system/uploads/attachment_data/file/435512/MHA_Code_of_Practice.PDF

22. U. Grundmann. Chapter 48. Anaesthesia for electroconvulsive therapy. In *Essentials of Neuroanesthesia*. Elsevier.

23. Guidance on the use of electroconvulsive therapy. *NICE Guidelines TA59*, October 2009. www.nice.org.uk/guidance/ta59/chapter/1-Guidance

24. Depression in adults: Treatment and management. *NICE Guidelines 222*, June 2022, www.nice.org.uk/guidance/ng222/chapter/Recommendations

25. Statement on Neurosurgery for Mental Disorder (NMD), also known as Psychiatric Neurosurgery. *Royal College of Psychiatrists*, February 2017, www.rcpsych.ac.uk/docs/default-source/about-us/who-we-are/ectcommittee-vns-dbs-ablative-neurosurgery-statement-feb17.pdf?sfvrsn=eba0287a_2

26. Ablative neurosurgery for obsessive compulsive disorder. *National Hospital for Neurology and Neurosurgery* (Patient Information Leaflet), https://advancedinterventions.org.uk/files/ACING_for_OCD_PIL.pdf

27. Repetitive transcranial magnetic stimulation for depression. *Nice Guidance 542*, www.nice.org.uk/guidance/ipg542

28. Statement on repetitive transcranial magnetic stimulation for depression. *Royal College of Psychiatrists*, February 2017, www.rcpsych.ac.uk/docs/default-source/about-us/who-we-are/ectcommittee-repetative-transcranial-magnetic-stimulation-statement-may18.pdf?sfvrsn=695e93be_2

29. Neuromodulation. *Royal College of Psychiatrist Leaflet*, www.rcpsych.ac.uk/mental-health/treatments-and-wellbeing/neuromodulation

30. Paul Harrison, Philip Cowen, Tom Burns, Mina Fazel. Chapter 5. Aetiology. In *Shorter Oxford textbook of psychiatry*, 7th edition. Oxford University Press.

31. Virginia L. Valentin, Nicole Mortier. *Population Health. Ballweg's physician assistant: A guide to clinical practice*, 7th edition. Oxford University Press.

32. Mental Capacity Act 2005. *UK Government*, www.legislation.gov.uk/ukpga/2005/9/contents

33. Mental Capacity and deprivation of liberty safeguards. *Newham Council*, www.newham.gov.uk/health-adult-social-care/mental-capacity-deprivation-liberty-safeguards
34. Lasting power of attorney, acting as an attorney. *Gov.UK*, www.gov.uk/lasting-power-attorney-duties
35. Human rights act 1998. *UK Government*, www.legislation.gov.uk/ukpga/1998/42/contents
36. Elizabeth Templeton, Richard William Kerslake, Lisanne Stock. *Revision guide for MRCPsych paper A*, 1st edition. Routledge.
37. Exploring mental health inpatient capacity across sustainability and transformation partnerships in England. *Royal College of Psychiatrists*, November 2019. Exploring mental health inpatient capacity across sustainability and transformation partnerships in England – Social Care Online (scie-socialcareonline.org.uk).
38. HelpGuide.org. How personality can impact your mental health. *Personality Types, Traits, and How It Affects Mental Health*. Accessed 19/07/2023

3　General adult psychiatry

Elijah Casper-Blake

Unipolar depression

Epidemiology[1–3]

- Prevalence estimated at 3.3% in England.
- Lifetime prevalence estimates vary ~4–30%.
- F:M ratio 2:1.
- Average age of onset mid to late 20's.

Aetiology[2,3,7]

- Genetics – Adoption studies and twin studies; 3x risk if present in a first-degree relative, hereditability ~37%.
- Childhood life experiences – Neglect and abuse, poor attachment relationships, parental depression.
- Psychological theories – Cognitive and behavioural ideas: Beck's model of depression, cognitive distortions, learned helplessness; Freud: mourning and melancholia.
- Neuroendocrine – Serotonin hypothesis, noradrenaline, dopamine, hypothalamic-pituitary-adrenal (HPA) axis changes (cortisol and thyroid function abnormalities).
- Neuroimaging – Enlarged ventricles, decreased hippocampal volume, white matter hyperintensities.
- Physical health problems – Often linked either due to their impact or as a result of medication, either directly (e.g., hypothyroidism, Cushing's) or indirectly (e.g., chronic pain and other comorbid physical health problems).
- Stressful life events – Studies suggest high frequency of stressful life events prior to the onset of depression.

DOI: 10.4324/9781003376163-3

Presentation[2,3,4,7]

- Core symptoms.

  - Low mood.
  - Anhedonia – Lack of enjoyment.
  - Anergia – Lack of energy.

- Cognitive symptoms.

  - Loss of self-esteem.
  - Feelings of guilt.
  - Feelings of worthlessness.
  - Negative thoughts.
  - Disrupted memory.
  - Poor concentration.

- Biological symptoms.

  - Loss of appetite.
  - Weight loss.
  - Lack of or disturbed sleep.
  - Loss of sexual desire.
  - Somatic symptoms.

- Other.

  - Agitation.
  - Slowing in cognitive processes, speech and motor movements.
  - Anxiety.
  - Psychotic symptoms – Symptoms can be wide-ranging but typically include mood congruent delusions, nihilistic delusions.

- Symptoms are generally present for at least 2 weeks.
- Symptoms should have an impact on an individual's functioning.

Management[5,6]

Mild depression

- Consider watchful waiting and further review in 2–4 weeks.
- Psychotherapy and social intervention are the first line of intervention.

  - Guided self-help.
  - Group exercise.
  - Mindfulness and meditation.
  - Counselling.
  - Cognitive behavioural therapy (CBT).

- Medication should not be routinely offered as first-line management for mild depression.

Moderate to severe

- Treatment depends on the individual's preference and can include either social and psychological interventions, medication or a combination of both in those with severe depression.
- Psychological therapy.
  - CBT, interpersonal therapy.
  - Short-term psychodynamic therapy.
  - Counselling.
  - Behavioural activation.
- Group exercise.
- Guided self-help or individual problem solving.

Antidepressants and suicide

- In some individuals, antidepressants may be linked to increased risk of suicide and increased thoughts of suicide in the short term.
- The evidence around this is not clear cut.
- Individuals felt to be most at risk are adolescents and young adults.
- In the long term, treating depression is likely to reduce the risk of suicide and suicidal thoughts.

Medication

- Selective serotonin reuptake inhibitors (**SSRIs**) and serotonin–norepinephrine reuptake inhibitors (**SNRIs**) are recommended as first-line treatments.
- Individuals should be reviewed after 2 weeks if aged >18 and after 1 week if <18.
- Response is usually seen within **4 weeks** but can be earlier.
- Treatment should be carried out for a **minimum of 6 months** post-remission for those experiencing a first episode of depression; in those who have had more than 1 episode it is suggested that they are carried on for a minimum of **2 years.**
- Stopping antidepressants should be done slowly, and it is recommended to reduce the dose in smaller steps each time, e.g., 50% or 25% of the previous dose.

Special circumstances and other treatments

Psychotic depression

- Treatment with an antidepressant and an antipsychotic is recommended.
- Maudsley guidelines suggests a tricyclic antidepressant as the first-line intervention with an SSRI or SNRI as the second line[6].

- Antipsychotics suggested are olanzapine and quetiapine.
- Fluoxetine + olanzapine is a commonly used combination.

STAR*D

- STAR*D was a large clinical trial looking into treatment strategies for depression.
- It involved 4 stages of treatment, with those not achieving remission progressing to the next level.

    - Level 1: citalopram.
    - Level 2: either switch or augment to an alternate antidepressant/ CBT.
    - Level 3: switch to mirtazapine or nortriptyline or augment with lithium or T3.
    - Level 4 switch to mirtazapine + venlafaxine or tranylcypromine.

- The results showed that remission rates were around 27–33% at level 1, and that switching at level 2 saw a further 25% remission rate.
- No clear advantage was demonstrated for switching or augmenting.
- The total cumulative remission rate after all 4 levels was 67%.
- Remission rates after the first two levels were significantly lower.

Treatment-resistant depression

- Reassessment is vital – ensuring that the diagnosis is in fact depression.
- Management of any comorbid conditions, including substance misuse.
- Evaluation of previous treatment – including ensuring that optimum dosing has been achieved prior to stopping.
- Evaluation of any social or sustaining factors.
- Medication.

    - Consider swapping to or adding in an antidepressant of another class.
    - Augmentation with lithium or a second-generation antipsychotic (evidence for use in non-psychotic depression).
    - Lamotrigine.
    - NICE also lists tri-iodothyronine as a possibility.

- ECT.

Electroconvulsion therapy (ECT)

Indications for ECT in depression:

- In life threatening circumstances where a quick response is needed.

- Where other treatments have not been successful and an individual wishes to try ECT.
- Where ECT has been helpful in the past and is the choice of an individual.
- Please see Chapter 2: organisation and delivery of psychiatric services for full details about ECT.

Repetitive transcranial magnetic stimulation (rTMS)

- rTMS is a relatively new, non-invasive form of treatment for depression.
- NICE indicates that rTMS can be used as a treatment for depression.
- Please see Chapter 2: organisation and delivery of psychiatric services for full details about rTMS.

Ketamine

- Ketamine is an emerging treatment for those with severe or treatment-resistant depression.
- It is not currently recommended by NICE for treatment of depression due to concerns about its cost and effectiveness.
- Ketamine can be given either intravenously or as a nasal spray.
- Ketamine may need to be administered on multiple occasions to maintain its effectiveness.
- It has been suggested that ketamine could be used for a rapid response and may be used in place of ECT.
- Ketamine has a number of cardiovascular side effects and some patients report feelings of dissociation.

St John's wort

- St John's wort is a preparation from the ***Hypericum perforatum*** plant.
- There seems to be some evidence for its use in mild to moderate depression.
- St John's wort is an enzyme inducer (intestinal and liver) and can have significant drug interactions as a result.
- St John's wort is not recommended by NICE due to concerns that it is not standardised in the UK and the potency of individual preparations can vary.

Poor prognostic factors

- Previous depressive episodes.
- Lack of support structure.
- Ongoing complicating factors/social stressors.
- Poor treatment response.
- Physical health problems/chronic pain.
- Substance misuse.

Outcomes[2,3,7]

- Depressive episodes last on average 6 months but in many individuals can be longer.
- 80% of individuals who have 1 episode of depression will go on to have a further episode.
- 5–10% of individuals initially felt to be suffering with depression may go on to later be diagnosed with bipolar affective disorder.
- Having a history of depression increases the risk of suicide and self-harm 15 times compared to having no history of depression.
- Individuals with depression have poorer physical health outcomes.
- Comorbid mental health and substance misuse disorders are common.

Bipolar affective disorder[7,18,19]

Epidemiology

- Lifetime risk – 0.3–3.9%.
- Prevalence ~2%.
- 1:1 M:F ratio.
- Age of onset ~18–21.

Aetiology

- Genetics – 85% hereditability, likely polygenic inheritance; possible crossover with genes for schizophrenia.
- Early childhood experiences such as trauma and abuse.
- Neurotransmitters – Dopamine, glutamate.
- HPA axis – Cortisol.
- Neuroimaging – Reduced brain volume, changes in hippocampal volume, white matter changes.
- Precipitating factors for relapse – stress, lack of sleep, drugs such as anti-depressants and steroids, recreational drugs.

Mania

Mania is an episode of heightened mood that lasts at least 7 days.
    Symptoms can include:

- Heightened mood and euphoria.
- Mood lability.
- Irritability and aggression.
- Increased energy and often reduced sleep.

- Increased activity.
- Racing thoughts and speech (pressure of speech and flight of ideas).
- Grandiosity and increased self-esteem.
- Impulsivity and disinhibition.
- Psychotic symptoms.

Presentation[21,22]

There are many different ways in which bipolar affective disorder has been classified across the ICD and DSM. Generally speaking:

- Individuals with bipolar may experience a mix of manic or hypomanic episodes as well as episodes of depression or mixed affective states.
- Broadly, bipolar affective disorder can be divided into **bipolar type 1, bipolar type 2, cyclothymia** and **other bipolar affective disorders**.
- **ICD-10** lists bipolar type 2 under other bipolar affective disorders, whereas **ICD-11** has a separate section for bipolar type 2.

Bipolar affective disorder

- Condition where an individual may experience a mix of manic or hypomanic episodes and episodes of depressive or mixed affective states.
- This can be with or without psychotic symptoms.
- Can be subdivided into various bipolar affective disorder subtypes, notably type 1 and type 2.
- ICD-10 does not specifically describe bipolar type 2 (it categorises this into **F31.8**: Other bipolar affective disorders), but the DSM-5 and ICD-11 have individual definitions.

Mixed affective states

Mixed affective states are a mixture of both manic and depressive symptoms.

- Symptoms can either be present together at the same time or they may alternate between depressive and manic symptoms.
- Symptoms must be present every day, most of the day for a period of 2 weeks.

Bipolar type 1

- Individuals who have experienced at least 1 manic episode and in addition may have experienced further manic, depressive or mixed episodes.

- In **ICD-11**, individuals **can be diagnosed with bipolar after 1 episode** of mania or mixed affective state, however **ICD-10 requires at least 2 episodes**, 1 of which is either manic or hypomanic.

Hypomania

Hypomania results in elevated mood and symptoms that are similar to that of mania, though generally less severe.

- Hypomanic episodes last for a period of days.
- Symptoms are disruptive but not significant enough to cause impaired functioning.
- Psychotic symptoms are not present in hypomania.

Bipolar type 2

- Individuals who have experienced at least 1 hypomanic episode and at least 1 depressive episode.

Cyclothymia

- Individuals experience fluctuations in mood between depressive symptoms and hypomanic symptoms.
- The symptoms tend to be present the majority of the time for an individual.
- Crucially, these symptoms are either not severe or prolonged enough to be classified as either a depressive illness or a manic or hypomanic episode.

Treatment[19,20,23]

Medication

Sodium valproate

- Sodium valproate had previously been recommended in the 2014 NICE guidelines for the management of bipolar affective disorder.
- However, the Medicines and Healthcare Products Regulatory Agency (MHRA) issued a warning about the risks associated with its use in pregnancy and with women of childbearing age.
- As such, its use in woman under the age of 55 is discouraged before exploring alternatives and is subject to close monitoring and review.

Acute mania

- Antipsychotic medication is the first line for an acute manic episode, e.g., **haloperidol, quetiapine, risperidone** or **olanzapine**.
- Clinicians may consider adding lithium or a mood stabiliser if ineffective.
- If an individual is on lithium already, their lithium level should be checked.
- If an individual is on an antidepressant, its discontinuation should be considered.
- ECT can be used for individuals with severe mania that has not responded to the aforementioned treatments, or where an urgent response is required.

Acute depressive episode

- **Olanzapine, quetiapine** or **lamotrigine** can be helpful.
- If this is ineffective or an individual is already on 1 of these, clinicians may consider combining antipsychotics with fluoxetine or switching to lamotrigine.
- If an individual is already on lithium and this has been optimised, olanzapine or lamotrigine may be added.

Long-term management

- NICE recommends the use of **lithium** as first-line treatment for the long-term management of bipolar affective disorder.
- Alternatives to this include antipsychotics, either **olanzapine** or **quetiapine**.

Psychology and other interventions

- Family therapy.
- Individual therapy, such as CBT or interpersonal therapy.
- Group therapy.
- Education and occupational support.
- Addressing any comorbid drug or alcohol use.
- Family and caregiver support.

Outcomes

- 50% of individuals will experience a relapse within 1 year.
- 90% of individuals will experience further episodes, and the average number of lifetime episodes is 10.
- Over time, remission of symptoms between episodes may become less complete and symptoms may present a significant impact on day-to-day life.
- Comorbid conditions are common with BPAD, particularly anxiety and substance misuse.

- Individuals with BPAD often have poorer physical health outcomes, e.g., cardiovascular, metabolic and respiratory diseases.
- **15% of individuals with BPAD end their lives**.

Psychosis

Schizophrenia[24,25,27]

Epidemiology

- Lifetime prevalence for schizophrenia ~0.5–1%.
- Onset is usually between the ages of 15–54.
- F:M ratio 1:1.

Aetiology

- Genetics – 85% hereditability, 10x risk if present in first-degree relatives.
- Maternal obstetric complications – Viral infection, pre-eclampsia, low birth weight, emergency c-section.
- Higher paternal age.
- Winter birth.
- Ethnicity – Individuals from an Afro-Caribbean background and their children living in the UK have a 6.7x risk of schizophrenia compared to the general population; individuals and their children from an Asian background living in the UK have a 1.5x risk compared to the general population.
- Early life adversity and childhood trauma – ~3x risk.
- Migration – 3x risk in first generation offspring.
- Urban living – 2.4x risk.
- Neuroimaging – Enlarged ventricles, decreased brain volume, smaller hippocampus and thalamus, changes in grey and white matter pathways.
- Neurotransmitters.

  - Dopamine hypothesis – Dopamine agonists can induce psychotic symptoms, and dopamine antagonists appear to be antipsychotic. Functional imaging suggests increased dopamine receptors, receptor occupancy and dopamine production in parts of the brain.
  - Glutamate – N-methyl D-aspartic acid (NMDA) receptor antagonists can induce psychosis.
  - Serotonin – Hallucinogens are thought in part to impact serotonin; some antipsychotics appear also to impact 5HT2 receptors.

- Substance misuse – Substances can precipitate psychotic symptoms; cannabis usage may be associated with the likelihood of developing schizophrenia.
- Medications – Corticosteroids.

Schneider's first rank symptoms

- Auditory hallucinations.
- Thought withdrawal.
- Thought insertion.
- Thought broadcast.
- Thought interruption.
- Somatic hallucinations.
- Delusional perception.
- Feelings or actions experienced as made or influenced by external agents.

Presentation[28]

- Schizophrenia is typically and episodic condition that follows a course of relapse and remittance; however, there can be periods of continuous illness as well as progressive deficits.
- Individuals may present with prodromal symptoms that don't quite meet the criteria for a full psychotic illness. These individuals may be classed as **at-risk individuals**.
- **Kurt Schneider** described what are classified as the **first rank symptoms of schizophrenia**, which are seen as core symptoms in the diagnosis of schizophrenia – however, these symptoms are not always present and are not exclusive to schizophrenia.
- Schizophrenia is typically characterised by **positive symptoms** which are **prominent in acute episodes** and **negative symptoms** which can be **more prominent in the chronic phase** (although both can be present in the acute and chronic phases).
  - **Positive symptoms** – Paranoid ideas and delusions, hallucinations.
  - **Negative symptoms** – Flattened affect, anhedonia, decreased motivation, poverty of speech, social withdrawal.
  - These sit alongside **cognitive** and **behavioural symptoms** such as thought disorders, unusual behaviour, cognitive impairment.
- The DSM does not divide schizophrenia into separate subtypes, but ICD-10 lists 7, alongside "schizophrenia unspecified" and "other schizophrenia."

Management[26,29]

AT-RISK INDIVIDUALS

- Offer CBT +/- family intervention.
- Treat comorbid mental health or substance misuse conditions.

Paranoid schizophrenia	• Predominant positive symptoms of paranoid delusions and hallucinations (generally auditory).
	• Affect, speech and motor symptoms are less prominent.
Hebephrenic schizophrenia	• Prominent affective symptoms and thought disorder alongside unusual mannerisms and unpredictable behaviour.
	• Delusions and hallucinations are fragmentary and less prominent.
	• Thought to have a poorer prognosis.
	• Negative symptoms can develop quickly.
Catatonic schizophrenia	• Predominant psychomotor disturbance.
	• Episodes of motor excitement (extreme hyperactivity).
	• Episodes of stupor (lack of movement and response despite no disturbance in consciousness).
	• Motor disturbance (posturing, rigidity, waxy flexibility).
	• Automatic obedience.
Undifferentiated	• No 1 specific subtype.
Post-schizophrenia depression	• Depressive episode following an acute phase of schizophrenia.
	• Symptoms of schizophrenia must still be present, but less prominent than in an acute phase.
Residual schizophrenia	• Chronic phase of schizophrenia characterised by negative symptoms.
Simple schizophrenia	• Progressive development of negative symptoms of schizophrenia.
	• Not preceded by positive psychotic symptoms as in residual schizophrenia.

- Do not offer an antipsychotic.
- Regular monitoring of subthreshold symptoms for up to 3 years.

FIRST EPISODE OF PSYCHOSIS

- Referral to early intervention in psychosis services.
- Treat comorbid mental health or substance misuse conditions.
- Offer antipsychotic medication alongside family interventions and CBT.

MAINTENANCE

- Community mental health service multidisciplinary treatment team (MDT) input.

- Psychosocial interventions alongside medication management.
- Antipsychotics are the mainstay in management and prevention of further relapses in schizophrenia.

  - Most individuals will require long-term antipsychotic treatment to prevent further relapse.
  - Engagement with medication should be monitored and depot medication may be considered to optimise management.

- Individuals should have frequent physical health monitoring, including assessment of weight, body mass index (BMI), electrocardiogram (ECG) and blood tests to monitor for side effects and metabolic impacts of antipsychotics.

Medication

CHOICE OF MEDICATION

- The choice of medication should primarily be dictated by an individual's circumstances and preferences. This should take into account:

  - What has worked or helped before.
  - Any comorbid physical health conditions, e.g., cardiac disease, diabetes, Parkinson's disease.
  - Individual drug side effects such as weight gain, cardiovascular risk, extrapyramidal side effects, raised prolactin levels.
  - Individual preference.
  - Method of administration, e.g., oral, sublingual, depot.

- Baseline measurements should be taken prior to starting and at intervals of antipsychotic medication:

  - Weight and height.
  - ECG.
  - Heart rate and blood pressure.
  - Blood tests including HbA1C, fasting lipids, prolactin levels.
  - Signs and risk of any movement disorders.

TREATMENT-RESISTANT SCHIZOPHRENIA

- Treatment-resistant schizophrenia is generally considered to occur when an individual has **not responded** to **adequate doses** of **2 different antipsychotics, at least 1** of which is a **second-generation antipsychotic**.
- **Clozapine therapy** is recommended as the **first line** for **treatment-resistant schizophrenia**.

- **High-dose antipsychotics**
  - This refers to the prescription of doses above the British National Formulary (BNF) maximum.
  - There is no clear evidence to suggest greater efficacy than antipsychotic doses within BNF limits.
  - Side-effect burdens may be more significant.
  - **High-dose antipsychotics** are generally **not recommended**.

- Maudsley guidelines list various alternatives to clozapine in treatment-resistant schizophrenia which tend to have less evidence behind them, including a combination of different antipsychotic therapies or augmentation with mood stabilisers and antidepressants, alongside other medications such as non-steroidal anti-inflammatory drugs (NSAIDs), omega-3 fatty acids, oestrogens and memantine.

Depot medications

Currently available long-acting medications:

- Aripiprazole.
- Risperidone.
- Paliperidone.
- Flupenthixol.
- Zuclopenthixol.
- Fluphenazine.
- Piptiazine.
- Haloperidol.
- Olanzapine.

LONG-ACTING ANTIPSYCHOTICS

Long-acting or "depot" antipsychotics are administered intramuscularly.

Long-acting antipsychotic medication is thought to help reduce the risk of relapse, particularly in those who may not be engaging with the medication regimen.

They also provide closer contact with the treatment team who usually administers a depot medication, and can allow clearer monitoring of an individual's engagement with medication.

Psychosocial support

- Family and caregiver support – Psychoeducation, involvement in care planning, crisis support, family therapy.
- Peer support.

- Employment and educational support.
- Treatment of any comorbid conditions and substance misuse.
- Physical health interventions.
  - Annual physical health monitoring, e.g., weight, cardiovascular and metabolic health.
  - Smoking cessation support and advice.

Risk factors for poorer prognosis

- Male gender.
- Early age of onset.
- Increased duration of untreated psychosis.
- Prominent negative symptoms.
- Comorbid substance misuse.
- Family history of schizophrenia.
- Lack of support structure.
- Low premorbid IQ.
- Poor insight and medication engagement.

Outcomes

- 4 in 5 individuals will see some improvement with treatment and 1 in 5 will not experience a further episode in 5 years.
- Aesop study – At a 10-year follow-up, 23% had unremitting illness and 45% had been free of symptoms for at least 2 years.
- Individuals with schizophrenia die on average 15 years earlier than the general population.
- Lifetime risk of suicide is 5–10%; risk is highest at the start of the illness, following recent discharge from hospital, in individuals with affective symptoms and history of suicide.
- 1.6x risk of death from all causes.
- Increased risk of physical morbidity, e.g., diabetes, obesity, smoking related illness, cardiovascular illness.
- Substance misuse is commonly comorbid.

Other psychotic illnesses[27,30,31]

Schizoaffective disorder	• Schizoaffective disorder is characterised by the presence of both mood/affective symptoms as well as symptoms of schizophrenia. • Affective symptoms can include manic, depressive and mixed symptoms. • Prevalence of 0.32–1.1%.

- Schizoaffective disorder shares many of the aetiological characteristics of both bipolar affective disorder and schizophrenia.
- Management is similar to that of other psychosis, with antipsychotics playing a key role, but mood stabilisers are often considered.

Delusional disorder
- Delusional disorder is characterised by a persistent delusion or set of delusional beliefs that generally remain stable over a prolonged period.
- Individuals do not meet the criteria for diagnosis of schizophrenia and symptoms such as auditory hallucinations and delusional control are absent.
- Individuals tend to have limited insight into their condition.
- Erotomania and delusional/morbid jealousy would fit under this category.
- Prevalence 1–3/100,000.
- Delusional disorders are often treated with antipsychotics but can often be quite resistant to treatment, and engagement with medications is often limited.
- They may be associated with comorbid alcohol and substance use.
- Management should consider mitigating any risks to others, particularly in the case of erotomania and delusional jealousy.

Anxiety disorders[35,36,39]

Epidemiology[34]

Condition	12-month prevalence	Lifetime prevalence
Generalised anxiety disorder	3.1%	5.7%
Panic disorder	2.7%	4.7%
Agoraphobia without panic disorder	0.8%	1.4%
Specific phobia	8.7%	12.5%
Social anxiety disorder	6.8%	12.1%

Aetiology

- Genetics – Twin studies suggest a link between anxiety disorders and depression.
- Neuroimaging – Role of the ventrolateral prefrontal cortex and amygdala.
- Neurotransmitters – GABA, noradrenaline, serotonin pathways implicated.
- Early life experiences – Particularly those where people feel under threat. Attachment theories.
- Cognitive behavioural theories – Conditioning, negative reinforcement.

Presentation[37]

Anxiety is associated with both psychological symptoms and multiple body systems. Symptoms that are common to most anxiety disorders are listed herein.

- **Psychological** – Feelings of fear and dread, poor concentration, sensitivity to noise and stimuli, irritability, feeling of unreality (depersonalisation or derealisation).
- **Gastrointestinal (GI)** – nausea and vomiting, GI upset (diarrhoea, flatulence, frequency), dry mouth, abdominal discomfort, a lump in the throat.
- **Genitourinary** – urinary frequency, sexual dysfunction, amenorrhoea.
- **Cardiovascular** – palpitations, chest pain and discomfort, blushing.
- **Respiratory** – Breathlessness/difficulty breathing.
- **Other** – Tremor, sweating, headache, muscle tension, tinnitus, tingling sensations, poor sleep, nightmares.

There is a range of anxiety disorders, which are broadly categorised in the following table.

Generalised anxiety disorder	• This is a feeling of persistent anxiety and worry that can be seen as "free floating." It is not triggered by a specific circumstance but instead can reach into multiple areas of a person's life as well as their predictions for the future. • Can be frequently experienced with panic disorder, depression and other phobias.
Agoraphobia	• Agoraphobia relates to anxiety provoked by a variety of situations including public or crowded places, leaving the home, confined places or places that are hard for them to leave. • Generally, an individual will look to avoid these situations and may be free of anxiety when not in these situations. • Panic disorder is commonly seen together with agoraphobia.
Social phobia	• Social phobia relates to anxiety provoked by social situations, they often manifest with a "fear of scrutiny" or being judged by others. • They can be more generalised, relating to all social situations, or more specific to actions such as public speaking. • These situations cause significant distress to the individual and often lead to avoidance, impacting multiple areas of an individual's life.
Specific phobias	• Anxiety provoked by a specific thing, e.g., spiders, heights, dogs, flying. • Anxiety is generally absent when an individual is not in contact with their specific phobia but can be provoked by images as well as imagination of that specific phobia.
Panic disorder	• Severe anxiety which occurs in frequent "attacks," often presenting with significant autonomic arousal symptoms (e.g., heart palpitations, breathlessness/hyperventilation, sweating, dizziness) alongside feelings of loss of control or feelings of impending doom.

Treatment[28]

GENERALISED ANXIETY DISORDER

- Step 1 – assessment and psychoeducation.
- Step 2 – Low intensity interventions: provide the individual with a self-help programme, this can be either in the form of resources or facilitator-guided individual or group self-help based around CBT principles.
- Step 3 – High-intensity psychological intervention such as CBT or applied relaxation or offer medication.
- Step 4 – Combination of high-intensity psychological interventions and medication.

Medication

SSRIs (sertraline) for first-line treatment; SNRIs are considered second-line treatment.

Pregabalin is licensed in the treatment of generalised anxiety disorder but would generally only be prescribed by a specialist.

Benzodiazepines should not be used except for a short-term crisis, and antipsychotic medication should not be prescribed.

PANIC DISORDER

First-line treatment is psychological therapy (CBT); however, if the disorder is longstanding or the individual has declined psychologically, then a medication can be offered (SSRI or SNRI).

SPECIFIC PHOBIA

Psychological intervention is the treatment of choice for specific phobias (CBT, exposure therapy) and medication is unlikely to play a significant role in its management.

SOCIAL PHOBIA

First-line treatment is psychological therapy (CBT); however, in cases where such interventions have been declined or been found ineffective, medication can be offered in the form of an SSRI (citalopram or fluvoxamine). If this is unsuccessful, another SSRI or venlafaxine (SNRI) may be considered.

AGORAPHOBIA

First-line treatment is psychological therapy (CBT, exposure therapy); however, medication can be offered similarly to other anxiety disorders, with SSRIs as first-line treatment and then SNRIs.

Outcomes

- Anxiety disorders often follow a chronic course, with those who have had a longer duration of symptoms more likely to be more significantly impacted.
- Anxiety disorders are frequently comorbid with other anxiety disorders, depression and substance misuse.
- Anxiety disorders can have a disabling impact on all areas of an individual's life.
- Psychological therapy has been shown to have an impact on anxiety disorders.
- 50% of those with generalised anxiety disorder who have remission of their symptoms will experience a further relapse.

Reactions to stress[35,40]

Acute stress reaction[37]

- Usually presents within minutes of an acutely stressful event and subsides within 2–3 days.
- Symptoms can present similarly to those of anxiety disorders. This includes autonomic arousal, narrowing of attention and consciousness, disorientation and daze-like feelings, agitation or a sense of numbness.
- An acute stress reaction, by definition, should resolve over a period of hours to days.

Adjustment reaction[37]

Adjustment disorder is an emotional and psychological response to a stressful circumstance or life event such as the loss of a job, change of school, loss of a partner or friend or illness. Adjustment disorders can present with depressive symptoms alongside feelings of anxiety and an inability to cope and can result in both distress and functional impairment.

Adjustment disorders usually resolve over a period of months. It may be appropriate for some individuals to offer counselling, problem solving or psychotherapy to help them to work through this change in circumstance.

Post-traumatic stress disorder (PTSD)[40,41]

Epidemiology

- The UK Adult Psychiatric Morbidity Survey found 31.4% of adults had experienced events that put themselves or persons close to them at risk of serious harm or death.
- 4.4% of all individuals screened positive for PTSD.

- Rates are highest for females aged 16–24 years old and reduce with age; for males, rates are relatively even between the ages of 16–64.
- Lifetime rates are estimated between 6–9%.
- Rates are higher in females.

Aetiology

- Stressful events.

    - By definition, an individual must have been involved in either directly or indirectly in a traumatic event.
    - Only 10% of individuals in such an event go onto develop PTSD.
    - Acts of violence and sexual assault are more likely than natural disasters to result in PTSD.
    - Previous trauma seems to increase the risk of PTSD.

- Comorbid mental health problems increase the risk of PTSD.
- Genetic – Twin studies suggest a genetic association.
- Neuroimaging – Amygdala hyperactivity, hippocampal atrophy.

Presentation[37]

- Symptoms generally present **within 6 months** of initial exposure to trauma (but can be delayed).
- Core symptoms:

    - **Re-experiencing** – Flashbacks, intrusive thoughts, nightmares.
    - **Avoidance** – Avoidance of triggers with links to the event, e.g., the area an event happened; this includes avoidance of thinking about the event and difficulty remembering details of the event.
    - **Hyperarousal** – Irritability, feeling of being constantly on edge and unable to relax, poor sleep, poor concentration.

- Other symptoms – Emotional numbing, decreased interest and enjoyment in activities, social withdrawal.
- Anxiety and depression alongside substance misuse can often be comorbid.

Treatment[42]

For those who experienced an acute stress disorder or who have significant PTSD symptoms following a trauma over the last month:

- Mild symptoms can be managed with active monitoring and review in 1 month's time.
- Trauma-focused CBT can be offered.
- Debriefing is not recommended.

For those with diagnosed PTSD or significant PTSD symptoms, the following can be offered:

- 8–12 sessions of **trauma-focused CBT**.
- Eye movement desensitisation and reprocessing (**EDMR**).
- Computerised or supported CBT.

Medication

- An SSRI such as **sertraline** or an SNRI (**venlafaxine**) may be offered if an individual wishes to start medication.
- Antipsychotics can be considered in those with severe symptoms such as psychosis or significant, disabling hyperarousal.
- **Benzodiazepines** should be **avoided.**

Outcomes

- PTSD symptoms can follow a fluctuant course.
- 40% of individuals may experience chronic symptoms.
- Other may achieve remission of their symptoms.

Obsessive-compulsive disorder (OCD)[35,36,43]

Epidemiology

- Population prevalence 1–3%.
- Lifetime prevalence around 1.5%.
- 1:1 M:F ratio
- Peaks in childhood and then again in early 20's.

Aetiology

- 3x risk if a relative has the disorder.
- Anatomy – Basal ganglia misfunction implicated.
- Autoimmune – Paediatric autoimmune neuropsychiatric disorder associated with *Streptococcus* (PANDAS).
- Psychoanalysis – repression, reaction formation, regression to the anal stage of development.

Presentation[37]

- **Obsessions**.
    - These are **intrusive** and repetitive thoughts, ruminations, images or urges that can be varied in nature and generally **cause distress** or feelings of anxiety in an individual.

- Common examples would be of religious imagery, violent images, fears of contamination or disastrous events, sexual imagery.
- **Compulsions**.
    - These are actions or thoughts that an individual feels that they must carry out.
    - They may include activity that is related to an individual's obsession, though it does not have to have a clear connection.
    - Examples might include checking, washing/cleaning, ordering of objects, specific rituals that an individual has to complete.
- Importantly, both obsessions and compulsions are felt to be of the **individuals own mind**, but they are generally **ego dystonic** and cause distress or anxiety.
- These obsessions and compulsions **must** either **cause significant distress**, have an **impact on an individual's day-to-day life** or **take >1 hour a day**.

Treatment[44]

Mild OCD

- Low intensity psychotherapy.
- Exposure and response prevention.
- Brief individual or group CBT.

Moderately severe OCD

- Intensive CBT or an SSRI.

Severe OCD

- Intensive CBT and an SSRI.

Treatment-resistant OCD

- Clomipramine.
- Buspirone and an SSRI.
- Augmentation with an antipsychotic.
- Neurosurgery is not recommended by NICE but can be considered in those with severe treatment-resistant symptoms upon request.

Outcomes

- 2 in 3 individuals improve in 1 year.
- Psychological therapy is effective at reducing symptoms – CBT causes an improvement in 60–80% of individuals.

- OCD can significantly impact an individual's quality of life and level of daily functioning,
- Risk of self-harm and suicide are increased.

Body dysmorphic disorder (BDD)[36,44]

Body dysmorphic disorder is a diagnosis that is part of hypochondrial disorder in ICD-10 but is a separate entity in the DSM.

Presentation

- Around 0.5–0.7% of the population has BDD.
- A preoccupation with what is perceived to be a significant problem or defect in an individual's appearance which to others is not perceived to be significant.
- Felt to be an overvalued idea.
- Commonly impacts the nose and ears but can impact any area of the body.
- Affected individuals may go to some lengths trying to camouflage or hide the perceived defect.
- Avoidance of social contact is common.
- Individual may seek out plastic surgery, though this often does not result in the resolution of symptoms.

Treatment

- Comorbid mental health conditions should be reviewed.
- Any acute risks of harm to self should be considered.
- Joint work with dermatologists and plastic surgeons can be helpful.
- For mild symptoms, CBT can be offered.
- For moderate symptoms, an SSRI (fluoxetine) or intensive CBT can be used.
- For severe symptoms, intensive CBT and an SSRI should be offered.

Somatisation disorders[32,37,45]

Hypochondriasis	• Prevalence 0.8–2.2%.
	• Presents with a preoccupation that an individual may be suffering from a significant medical illness despite reassurances from medical professionals.
	• Often comorbid with anxiety and depression.
	• May be linked to an altered interpretation of bodily sensations or selective attention.
Somatisation disorder	• F:M ratio 10:1
	• Individuals present with recurrent symptoms that can stretch across a range of bodily systems.
	• These symptoms are not found to have an underlying cause.
	• Symptoms can change or shift to other areas over time.
	• Individuals will often have had a significant number of medical referrals and investigations.

Conversion disorder	• Prevalence 50/100,000. • As much as 20% of outpatient neurology referrals. • Often begins before the age of 35. • Individuals present with unexplained neurological symptoms. • Symptoms can include isolated weaknesses, tremors, cognitive complaints, non-epileptic seizures.
Pain syndromes	• Individuals may experience persistent pain for which no underlying cause has been found. • There are specific pain syndromes relating to different parts of the body. • Presentation may vary dependent on the site of the pain. • There may be some evidence for the use of antidepressant medications in these conditions.

Management[32,45]

* Involves working closely with medical professionals looking to:

    * Minimise medical investigations and referrals.
    * Provide psychoeducation regarding the body-mind links.

* Focus on an individual's goals for rehabilitation.
* Consider physiotherapy input where appropriate (particularly in conversion disorder).
* Treat any comorbid depression or anxiety.
* Consider CBT or psychotherapy.

Malingering[32]

Malingering is the feigning of symptoms of an illness, generally in order to receive some form of secondary gain, e.g., seeking compensation in an accident, trying to avoid a situation.

Factitious disorder[32]

Factitious disorder is listed in the DSM and is the intentional production of symptoms or illness generally in order to receive medical care. The underlying causes of this are varied and may include a previous history of abuse, early life illness or familial illness, comorbid mental health conditions.

Munchausen's by proxy is a form of factitious illness where a parent or caregiver produces symptoms in another, often a child (but may also be an adult).

Dissociative disorders[32,37]

* Dissociative disorders are characterised by "a complete loss of the normal integration between memories of the past, awareness of identity and immediate sensations, and control of bodily movements."

- Presentations are varied, with ICD-10 classifying conversion disorders (mentioned earlier) within the same category.
- Dissociation is often thought of as a trauma response, and childhood abuse is felt to be a significant factor in its aetiology.

Dissociative amnesia	• Loss of memory, often around a recent significant or traumatic event, e.g., a car accident. • Amnesia is usually partial and centred around a specific event. • This loss of memory is not otherwise explained by organic cognitive impairment or by normal forgetfulness.
Dissociative fugue	• This is characterised by a loss of memory of events. • However, during a period of fugue, the individual may often travel some distance or engage in activities outside their normal routines. • Examples might include an individual travelling across the country and being unaware how they got there. • Individuals appear to be functioning normally to those on the outside. • In the DSM, this diagnosis is part of dissociative amnesia.
Dissociative stupor	• Individuals present as mute and unresponsive to their surroundings. • There is reduced movement. • Individuals remain conscious and aware. • Can be triggered by traumatic event. • Organic brain disease or other mental health conditions such as schizophrenia must be ruled out.
Dissociative identity disorder or multiple personality disorder	• Individuals present with 2 or more distinct identities. • Each identity has their own range of emotions and behaviours that can be quite different from one another. • Importantly, the individual identities are experienced as distinct identities separate from one another and from the self. • There is generally amnesia of events between identities, which leads to people feeling they have lost time.
Depersonalisation–derealisation disorder	• Individuals may experience feelings of detachment from the present moment. • They may feel that their thoughts or surroundings are unreal or that their body is on autopilot. • Individuals are aware of what is going on around them and fully conscious of events. • Depersonalisation-derealisation may be present in other conditions. • It is classified alongside dissociative disorders in the DSM but separately in ICD-10.
Other dissociative disorders	• Trance and possession disorder – Loss of sense of the self and awareness of surroundings, individuals are in a "trance-like" state. • Ganser's syndrome – Clouding of consciousness, nonsensical or approximate answers given to questions (**vorbeireden**), hallucinations/pseudohallucinations, somatic symptoms.

Personality disorders[46,47]

Epidemiology[48,49]

- Estimates of the prevalence of personality disorders vary. The UK Adult Psychiatric Morbidity Survey 2014 found:
  - **Any personality disorder – 13.7%.**
  - **Antisocial personality disorder – 3.3%.**
  - **Borderline personality disorder – 2.4%.**
- Exact prevalence rates for individual personality disorders vary from study to study; however, the **most common** appear to be **obsessive-compulsive, paranoid, borderline, histrionic** and **avoidant** personality disorders.
- The prevalence of personality disorder in psychiatric **inpatients can be up to 40%** and **up to 50% of individuals in prison** may have a personality disorder.
- Personality develops through childhood and adolescence, so personality disorders are not generally diagnosed until adulthood.

Aetiology

- Genetics – Twin studies suggest hereditability in antisocial personality disorder, borderline personality disorder and schizotypal personality disorder.
- Neurotransmitters – Monoamine oxidase and 5-HT receptors may play a role in antisocial behaviour.
- Early life experiences – Trauma, neglect and abuse, childhood behavioural difficulties (conduct disorder).
- Attachment theories, social learning theories.

Presentation[50,51]

- Personality is developed through childhood and relates to a broad range of traits that make up an individual's character.
- An individual's personality may impact the way that an individual sees themselves or interacts with those around them and their environment.
- Personality tends to be seen as:
  - Enduring – Personality traits tend to be fairly stable through life.
  - Pervasive – Personality has impacts on all areas of an individual's life.

Personality disorder

- Characterised by problems with:
  - An individual's **sense of self** – e.g., an individual's sense of self identity or worth.

- **interpersonal functioning** – An individual's ability to make and maintain relationships.

- These problems should cause significant impacts on multiple areas of an individual's life.
- They should have lasted for at least 2 years.
- They cannot be explained by any developmental or other conditions.

The classification of personality disorders is changing:

- ICD-11 no longer lists individual personality disorders (except for border-line personality disorder, which remains).
- Instead, an individual is diagnosed with either mild, moderate or severe severity personality disorder.
- A dimensional approach is used, with 5 individual domains that may be prominent for an individual.
- Following is a summary of the prominent traits for the individual personality disorder subtypes as used in ICD-10/DSM-5.

ICD-11 domains

- Negative affectivity – Emotional lability, difficulties regulating emotions, negative self-image and low self-esteem, frequent and intense negative emotions, mistrustfulness and suspicion.
- Detachment – Social detachment (limited social interactions and relationships), emotional detachment (limited range of emotions expressed, generally aloof and reserved).
- Dissociality – Self-centredness and lack of empathy for others.
- Disinhibition – impulsivity, distractibility, irresponsibility, reckless-ness, lack of planning.
- Anankastia – Perfectionism, emotional and behavioural constraint (rigidity and risk avoidance)

Treatment[52]

- Management of a personality disorder is likely to require a holistic approach.
- Full diagnostic assessment is needed alongside consideration of the impact that the condition may be having on an individual's life.
- Understanding each individual's perspective on their diagnosis and for-mulating personalised treatment goals is important.
- Consideration and treatment of any comorbid conditions such as anxiety, depression and substance misuse may be helpful.

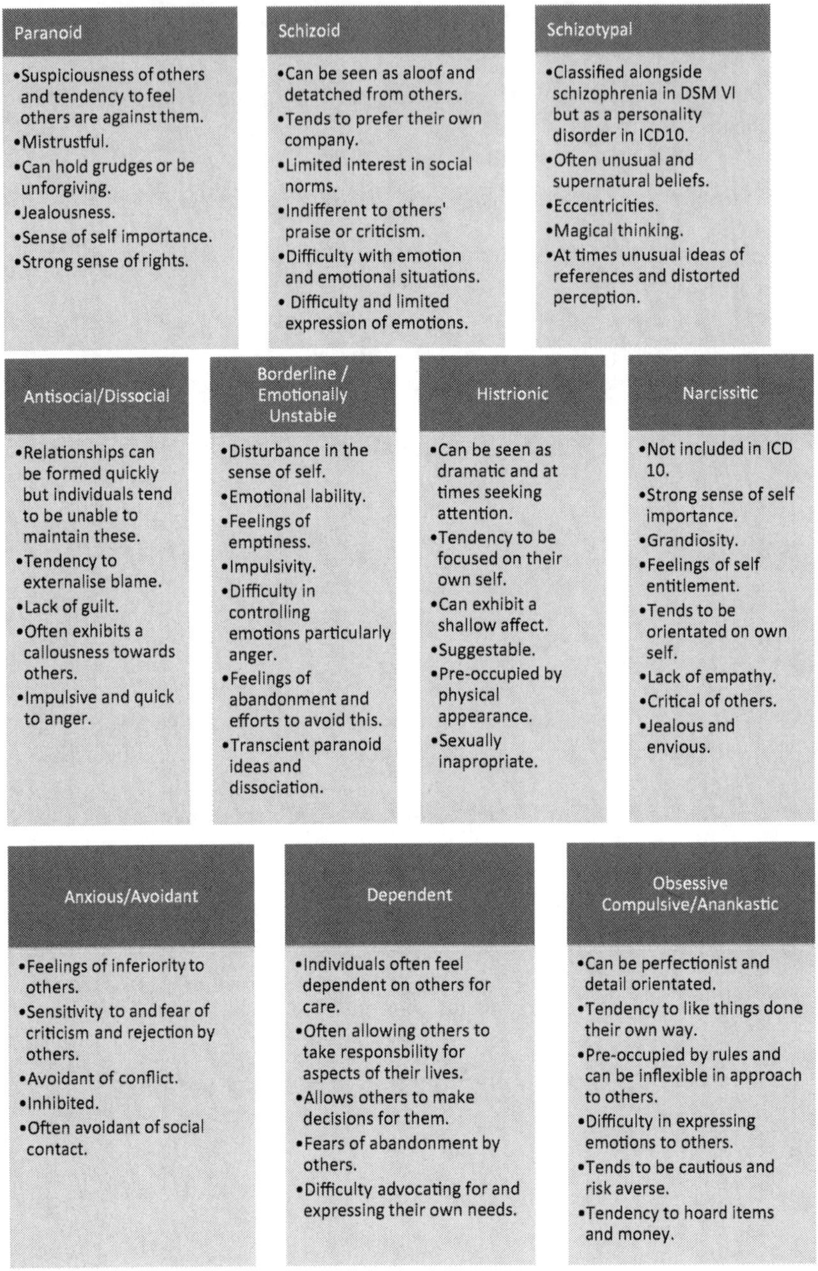

Paranoid

- Suspiciousness of others and tendency to feel others are against them.
- Mistrustful.
- Can hold grudges or be unforgiving.
- Jealousness.
- Sense of self importance.
- Strong sense of rights.

Schizoid

- Can be seen as aloof and detatched from others.
- Tends to prefer their own company.
- Limited interest in social norms.
- Indifferent to others' praise or criticism.
- Difficulty with emotion and emotional situations.
- Difficulty and limited expression of emotions.

Schizotypal

- Classified alongside schizophrenia in DSM VI but as a personality disorder in ICD10.
- Often unusual and supernatural beliefs.
- Eccentricities.
- Magical thinking.
- At times unusual ideas of references and distorted perception.

Antisocial/Dissocial

- Relationships can be formed quickly but individuals tend to be unable to maintain these.
- Tendency to externalise blame.
- Lack of guilt.
- Often exhibits a callousness towards others.
- Impulsive and quick to anger.

Borderline / Emotionally Unstable

- Disturbance in the sense of self.
- Emotional lability.
- Feelings of emptiness.
- Impulsivity.
- Difficulty in controlling emotions particularly anger.
- Feelings of abandonment and efforts to avoid this.
- Transcient paranoid ideas and dissociation.

Histrionic

- Can be seen as dramatic and at times seeking attention.
- Tendency to be focused on their own self.
- Can exhibit a shallow affect.
- Suggestable.
- Pre-occupied by physical appearance.
- Sexually inapropriate.

Narcissitic

- Not included in ICD 10.
- Strong sense of self importance.
- Grandiosity.
- Feelings of self entitlement.
- Tends to be orientated on own self.
- Lack of empathy.
- Critical of others.
- Jealous and envious.

Anxious/Avoidant

- Feelings of inferiority to others.
- Sensitivity to and fear of criticism and rejection by others.
- Avoidant of conflict.
- Inhibited.
- Often avoidant of social contact.

Dependent

- Individuals often feel dependent on others for care.
- Often allowing others to take responsbility for aspects of their lives.
- Allows others to make decisions for them.
- Fears of abandonment by others.
- Difficulty advocating for and expressing their own needs.

Obsessive Compulsive/Anankastic

- Can be perfectionist and detail orientated.
- Tendency to like things done their own way.
- Pre-occupied by rules and can be inflexible in approach to others.
- Difficulty in expressing emotions to others.
- Tends to be cautious and risk averse.
- Tendency to hoard items and money.

Figure 3.1 The 10 different personality disorders

- Most localities will have their own specialist personality disorder services, but individuals may also be managed in community mental health teams.
- **Psychological therapy is the mainstay of treatment** for personality disorders, with the most evidence for the treatment of borderline personality disorder.
  - **Schema therapy.**
  - **Mentalisation-based therapy.**
  - **Dialectical behavioural therapy.**
  - **Transference-based psychotherapy.**

Medication

Although medication is frequently used in practice, NICE does not recommend the use of medication for personality disorder unless there are comorbid mental health conditions.

Outcomes

- Questions remain regarding the course of personality disorders; however, its generally felt that individual traits may wax and wane in prominence through an individual's life and depending on their current circumstances.
- Some studies have shown that 50% of individuals reassessed later in life no longer fit the criteria for personality disorder.
- Comorbidity with personality disorder is common.
- The long-term risk of suicide in individuals with personality disorder is high, particularly in individuals with borderline personality disorder (10%).

Assessment and management of disorders related to pregnancy and childbirth

Antenatal and postnatal depression[32,53,54]

Postnatal mood disturbance

- Commonly called "the baby blues."
- Felt to be a normal part of pregnancy.
- Experienced by 50–75% of mothers.
- More common in first pregnancies.
- Symptoms include feeling confused, lability in mood – often alternating between happiness and feeling miserable, episodes of crying and irritability.
- Can last for several days after giving birth but will resolve spontaneously.
- Does not require treatment.

Epidemiology

- 12% of woman are thought to suffer from depression during the course of pregnancy.
- 15–20% of woman may experience depression in the year following giving birth.
- Many of those individuals who are diagnosed with postnatal depression had symptoms that began prior to the birth of their child.

Presentation

- Presentation may be similar to that of general depression; however, anxiety, irritability and tiredness may be more prominent. Alongside this, there may be feelings of guilt and fears of harm coming to their baby.
- Onset is usually thought to occur within 4 weeks to a year of having a baby.
- Can be screened for using the **Edinburgh Post-Natal Depression Scale.**

RISK FACTORS

- Previous history of depression or pregnancy-related depression.
- Having had "the baby blues."
- Younger age.
- Marital difficulties.
- History of domestic violence.
- Lack of social support.
- Life stress.
- Unplanned pregnancy.
- Unemployment.
- Having had previous children.
- Infant health complications.

Management

MILD TO MODERATE

- Psychological intervention or facilitated self-help.
- If there is a history of severe depression, then antidepressant medication can be considered.

MODERATE TO SEVERE DEPRESSION

- High-intensity psychological therapy, e.g., CBT.

- Medication SSRI, SNRI, tricyclic antidepressants.
- Or a combination of both.

Prognosis

- Depression may subside over a period of months.
- 1 in 3 women will continue to experience depressive symptoms after 1 year.
- Depression can have a significant impact on mother–baby bonding, along with family and partner relationships.
- Untreated depression may have an impact on infant failure to thrive, alongside increased risk of childhood mental illness such as depression.

Puerperal psychosis[32,53]

SUMMARY

- Incidence is around 1/500–1/1000 pregnancies.
- Family history of bipolar affective disorder.
- Personal history of bipolar affective disorder (20% relapse risk during pregnancy).
- Onset is usually within 2 weeks of delivery.
- Symptoms come on rapidly
- Symptoms represent affective psychosis similar to bipolar affective disorder.
- Fluctuating course.
- Other presentations described are "delirium" and "schizophreniform" types, though these are thought to be less common.

Management

- Referral to specialist services.
- Immediate assessment of risk to both mother and baby.
- Many affected individuals are likely to require a period of hospitalisation for treatment.
- First-line medications are **antipsychotics**.

Prognosis

- Most individuals recover well from an episode of puerperal psychosis.
- Affected individuals have a ~50% risk of further episodes in subsequent pregnancies.
- Some individuals may go on to suffer from bipolar affective disorder.

General principles of managing mental illnesses during pregnancy[56,57]

- Involvement of the mother/parents in all decision making.
- Consideration of non-pharmacological approaches where applicable.
- Acknowledgement of the baseline risks of foetal malformation and miscarriage for all pregnancies.
- Acknowledgement of the risks that all medications may pose.
- Acknowledgement that we do not have a complete set of safety data for most medications in pregnancy.
- Discussion of the risks of relapse and the risks associated with not treating a mental illness for both the mother and baby, assessing an individual's past psychiatric history.
- Awareness of the risks of relapse if medication is abruptly stopped.
- Use of the safest medications at the minimum effective doses possible.
- Consideration of medication that has been helpful for the individual in the past alongside the risks and benefits of switching to alternatives.
- Consideration for referral to specialist services where appropriate.

Specific conditions in pregnancy[19,25,55,56]

Anxiety	• Psychotherapy is the first-line treatment for anxiety.
	• If an individual is on medication, it may be appropriate to consider whether this is still required.
	• Medication is not specifically recommended but may be appropriate in individuals with severe symptoms.
	• Antidepressant medication may be appropriate if required, typically an SSRI or TCA.
Alcohol and substance misuse	• Referral to specialist drug and alcohol services is appropriate.
	• Additional input from perinatal services and co-operation with obstetricians are likely to be beneficial.
	• Harm reduction methods are recommended.
	• Considerations can be made dependant on the individual substance of concern and the benefit of detoxification or substitute medication.

Eating disorders	• Psychotherapy is the first-line intervention. • Close monitoring of mental state in the pre- and post-natal periods is recommended. • Specific advice and consideration may need to be given regarding maternal diet, alongside feeding support.
Bipolar affective disorder	• Individuals should be referred to specialist perinatal services. • Discussion should be had around the risks and benefits of remaining on a current medication, stopping or reducing dose or switching to another medication, particularly for those on **lithium** or **mood stabilisers**. • There is a high risk of relapse during or following pregnancy (up to **60% relapse rate** in the first 3 months post-birth). • Antipsychotic medication is considered the first line for pro-phylaxis and treatment of bipolar affective disorder during pregnancy.
Schizophrenia	• Individuals should be referred to specialist perinatal services. • Discussion should be had of the risks and benefits of remaining on current medication, stopping or reducing dose or switching to another medication. • It is generally recommended that medication should be continued throughout pregnancy due to the risks of untreated schizophrenia. • Antipsychotics are the first line in the treatment for acute psychosis or schizophrenia.

Specific medications[19,25,54–58]

USE DURING PREGNANCY

It is difficult to complete safety trials of medication in pregnancy. As a result, much of the data we have on the safety of psychotropic medication can be complicated by various factors.

When discussing specific medications with service users it can be helpful to use resources such as the **Maudsley Prescribing Guide** or the **Best Use of Medicines in Pregnancy (BUMPS)** website by the UK Teratology Information Service. These resources provide a detailed summary of the data we have for individual medications in pregnancy.

Antidepressants	• Generally, there is a higher threshold for prescribing antidepressants in pregnancy.
	• **Sertraline** is recommended by the Maudsley guidelines as first-line treatment.
	• Other sources suggest using **fluoxetine** or a **TCA**, as these have the most safety data.
	• **SSRIs**
	• SSRIs do not appear to be majorly teratogenic.
	• **Paroxetine** may have an association with **cardiac malformations**.
	• Possible link to low birth weight, pre-term delivery and spontaneous miscarriage.
	• **SSRIs** may be associated with an increased risk of **post-partum haemorrhage**.
	• **TCAs**
	• TCAs are not thought to be generally teratogenic.
	• **Clomipramine** may be linked to **cardiac defects**.
	• Possibly linked to pre-term delivery, pre-eclampsia and spontaneous miscarriage.
	• **SNRIs**
	• **Venlafaxine** may be associated with **cardiac defects, anencephaly** and **cleft palate**, although this link is not clear.
	• **MAOIs** – Avoid the use of MAOIs due to the risk of malformations.
	• All antidepressants have a risk of **neonatal discontinuation symptoms**; these tend to be mild and self-limiting but can result in irritability, lethargy, low Apgar scores and respiratory or neurological symptoms (such as convulsions).
	• **SSRIs** and **SNRIs** increase the risk of **persistent pulmonary hypertension,** though the risk of this is low.
Antipsychotics	• Neither first- nor second-generation antipsychotics are felt to be major teratogens.
	• Some studies do show increased risks regarding antipsychotic use during pregnancy, but further study may be helpful.
	• Be aware of the endocrine and metabolic side effects of antipsychotics, e.g., weight gain, increased diabetes risk and hyperprolactinaemia.
	• **Antipsychotic discontinuation** symptoms may occur in infants following birth – increased crying, agitation and suckling.
	• Maudsley guidelines recommend using either **quetiapine, olanzapine, risperidone** or **haloperidol**.
	• Additional monitoring and dietary advice may be recommended.
Lithium	• Lithium should generally be avoided in those seeking to become pregnant unless considered necessary due to concerns around risks or other treatments being ineffective.
	• In those already on lithium or for whom lithium may be the best treatment, the risks and benefits of continuing lithium treatment at the lowest effective dose should be considered.
	• There is a high (~70%) risk of relapse post-partum if lithium is stopped.
	• Lithium is associated with cardiac malformation, particularly Epstein's anomaly (10x risk). The risk is highest following exposure to lithium between 2–6 weeks of pregnancy.

	• Risks to the baby include hypothyroidism, post-delivery lethargy, hypotonia. • In individuals who opt to continue lithium during pregnancy, increased lithium monitoring is advised. Increased ultrasound monitoring during pregnancy may also be offered.
Other mood stabilisers	• Recommendations are to generally avoid the use of mood stabilising drugs during pregnancy in preference of antipsychotic medications. • Treatment should not be stopped abruptly, and support from specialist services should be sought. • **Sodium valproate has a ~10%** risk of major malformations. • **Carbamazepine** and **sodium valproate** both confer an increased risk of neural tube defects. • **Sodium valproate** confers an increased risk of spina bifida, cleft palate, hypospadias, polydactylism, craniosynostosis and cardiac septal defects. It has also been associated with low IQ in children exposed to it during pregnancy.
Benzodiazepines	• Benzodiazepines may be associated with **cleft lip, cardiac malformations** and **alimentary tract malformations**. • **Low birth weight** is a risk, along with **lethargy, floppy baby syndrome**, and a need for **respiratory support** post-delivery. • Advice is to avoid usage, except for short-term use to manage severe symptoms.

Breastfeeding

Antidepressants	• Sertraline and mirtazapine are recommended • Fluoxetine and citalopram may accumulate in breast milk, and it may be best to avoid their use.
Antipsychotics	• Quetiapine and olanzapine are recommended. • Avoid breastfeeding with clozapine.
Lithium and mood stabilisers	• Avoid breastfeeding whilst on lithium and carbamazepine. • Antipsychotics should be used in favour of mood stabilisers if required.
Benzodiazepines	• Avoid where possible, and if used, then opt for drugs with a shorter half-life if necessary.

General hospital psychiatry

Delirium/acute confusional state[32]

Delirium is an acute disturbance of the mind, characterised by clouded consciousness, fluctuating confusion and reduced attention.

Delirium is multifactorial and can have a number of physical and physiological causes. It is most common in those individuals with increased frailty or conditions that impact the mind such as dementia, previous stroke or learning disabilities.

Delirium will be covered in detail in Chapter 4: Old Age Psychiatry.

Psychiatry and medical conditions[9,32]

CARDIOVASCULAR[59,60]

- Mental illness, alongside the use of many psychotropic medications, can be a risk factor for cardiovascular disease.
- Depression is felt to be an independent risk factor for cardiovascular disease, alongside anxiety. Screening for both these may be appropriate post myocardial infarction. **Sertraline** is the medication of choice.
- QTc interval – Many psychotropic medications, including most **antipsychotics**, some antidepressants (such as **citalopram**), other substances (such as **methadone**), can cause an increased QTc interval.

ENDOCRINE[61]

- Diabetes.
  - Diabetes often has a significant impact on an individual's life and can be a psychological stressor.
  - Diabetic control is likely to be impacted by psychological stress.
  - Hypoglycaemia may provoke feelings of anxiety.
  - Diabetes is a risk factor for vascular dementia.
  - 10–15% of individuals with diabetes may have depression.
  - Many psychotropic drugs have a risk of developing metabolic complications, e.g., **antipsychotics** and **mirtazapine**.
  - Insulin use – Individuals with an eating disorder may omit insulin in order to lose weight; some individuals may abuse insulin for self-harm or suicide.
- Thyroid disease.
  - Hyperthyroidism is associated with anxiety-type symptoms.
  - Hypothyroidism can be associated with depressive symptoms, dementia symptoms and rarely with psychosis and mania.
- Cortisol.
  - Excess cortisol, such as with corticosteroid use or in Cushing's syndrome, can be associated with confusion/delirium and depressive symptoms alongside mania.
  - Addison's disease (primary adrenal insufficiency) is also associated with depressive symptoms.
- Phaeochromocytoma – May be associated with anxiety and panic type symptoms.

HEPATIC AND RENAL IMPAIRMENT[62]

- Extra care must be taken when prescribing psychiatric medications to patients with hepatic or renal impairment.

- Advice or guidance should be sought regarding any medication prescribed to individuals with hepatic or renal impairment on a case-by-case basis.
- Dosage adjustments may be required depending on the medication.

	Hepatic impairment	*Renal impairment*
Antidepressants	Paroxetine, citalopram, sertraline, vortioxetine	Sertraline, citalopram, fluoxetine
Antipsychotics	Sulpride or amisulpride	Haloperidol or olanzapine, avoid sulpride and amisulpride
Mood stabilisers	Lithium	Sodium valproate or lamotrigine, avoid lithium
Sedatives	Shorter acting sedatives such as oxazepam, temazepam and lorazepam	Lorazepam

Neuropsychiatric consequences of physical health conditions[8–12,32]

Multiple sclerosis
- Multiple sclerosis is a condition that effects the central nervous system.
- The core pathology is the demyelination of sites within the brain.
- Its prevalence is around 60–100/100,000.
- Onset is usually between the ages of 20–45.
- Symptoms tend to follow a relapsing and remitting course for 80–90% of individuals; however, 10–20% follow a primary progressing course with others later going on to run a progressive course.
- Symptoms vary depending on the areas of the brain impacted.
- Drugs used in the treatment of multiple sclerosis (e.g., corticosteroids and interferons) may cause neuropsychiatric symptoms, as well as the condition itself.
- Neuropsychiatric symptoms can include:
  - Mood lability.
  - Fatigue.
  - Depression is 50% of individuals.
  - Increased risk of suicide.
  - Cognitive impairment.
  - Potential to develop dementia (60%).
  - Less frequently manic or psychotic symptoms.

Huntington's disease
- Huntington's disease is a form of progressive neurological disease that caused both chorea and dementia.
- It is an autosomal dominant condition which causes cerebral atrophy, particularly in the caudate and putamen, along with changes in the frontal lobe.
- Prevalence is 5/100,000.
- Neuropsychiatric symptoms are particularly common in Huntington's disease, and individuals may present with these symptoms early in the illness.
- Neuropsychiatric symptoms can include:
  - Depression (50% of affected individuals).
  - Increased suicide risk (10x that of the general population).
  - Irritability.
  - Apathy.
  - Impulsivity.
  - Cognitive slowing.
  - Schizophrenia-like psychosis (10% of affected individuals).

Parkinson's disease	• Parkinson's disease is a neurological condition characterised by symptoms of rigidity, tremor and bradykinesia.
	• Parkinson's pathology primarily results from degeneration of neurones within the substantia nigra and other areas of the basal ganglia. The development of Lewy bodies and the loss of dopaminergic neurons are seen.
	• Onset is usually around the age of 55.
	• Prevalence of 150/100,000.
	• Neuropsychiatric symptoms are common in Parkinson's disease and can be the direct result of the pathology as well as the medication given (e.g., dopamine and dopamine agonists).
	• Neuropsychiatric symptoms can include:
	• Depression in 45–58% of individuals.
	• Anxiety.
	• Apathy.
	• Cognitive impairment (around 80% of individuals will develop dementia after 8+ years of the condition).
	• Hallucinations (particularly visual) and psychotic symptoms are common (20–40% of affected individuals).
	• Sleep disorder – Particularly REM sleep disorder.
	• Impulse control disorders – May be medication-related.
Stroke	• Strokes are vascular events that lead to cerebral deficits or dysfunction. They are generally thought of as either **ischaemic** or **haemorrhagic** in nature.
	• 200 of every 100,000 individuals who have a stroke each year die.
	• Strokes are more common in males and older individuals.
	• The aetiology of strokes is varied, but vascular risk factors tend to play a significant role.
	• Neuropsychiatric symptoms can include:
	• Frontal lobe syndromes.
	• Apathy.
	• Irritability.
	• Mood lability, alongside extreme emotionality.
	• Depression in around 30–33% of affected individuals.
	• Cognitive impairment and vascular dementias.
Wilson's disease	• Wilson's disease is a condition that results from errors in copper metabolism
	• Individuals with Wilson's disease have abnormal deposits of copper that may be focused in the liver, resulting in hepatitis; in the eyes, resulting in **Kaiser-Fleischer rings**; or alongside deposits in the brain basal ganglia, often resulting in tremor and dysarthria.
	• Autosomal recessive condition.
	• Effects 1/30,000–1/100,000 individuals.
	• Neuropsychiatric symptoms can include:
	• Depression.
	• Personality change.
	• Psychotic symptoms.
Head injury	• Trauma to the head can lead to a variety of symptoms, depending on the mechanism involved and the extent and site of the injury.
	• Brain damage can occur as a result of **direct damage to neurones** from trauma, **shearing forces** of an accident and/or associated **hypoxia**, **ischaemia** and **oedema**.

- Acute symptoms can range from headache and periods of confusion to loss of consciousness with more severe head injuries.
- **Glasgow Coma Score** over time and assessment of **post-traumatic amnesia** are helpful in understanding the severity and prognosis of head injury.
- **Post-concussion syndrome**
  - Seen in 15–50% of individuals after mild head injury.
  - Has a broad range of neuropsychiatric symptoms, including mood disturbance, irritability, anxiety, poor sleep, poor concentration, headache and dizziness.
  - Symptoms generally resolve without a need for treatment.
  - Some individuals may experience for at least 1 year.
- Longer-term neuropsychiatric symptoms can be varied:
  - Personality changes are common with frontal lobe injuries – this can include reduced inhibitions, apathy, irritability, anger and aggression.
  - Delirium after head injury.
  - Cognitive impairment.
  - Depression and anxiety are common and seen in ~50% of affected individuals.
  - Some individuals may make a full recovery from mild injuries, but others may need longer-term support from rehabilitation with a specialist MDT.

Encephalitis
- Encephalitis refers to inflammation of the brain.
- Encephalitis is often **viral** (e.g., herpes simplex virus, Epstein-Barr virus, mumps) but can also relate to **bacterial** infections and **autoimmune** conditions.
- Symptoms can develop over a short time period (hours to days).
- Physical symptoms may include fever, headache, neurological signs, seizures and reduced levels of consciousness.
- Neuropsychiatric symptoms can include:
  - Personality change.
  - Anxiety.
  - Depression.
  - Delirium and confusion.
  - Psychotic symptoms have also been postulated.
- Diagnosis relies on clinical imaging alongside magnetic resonance imaging (MRI), lumber puncture and electroencephalography (EEG).

Epilepsy
- Epilepsy is condition characterised by recurrent seizures.
- It has a prevalence of 7/1000.
- Psychiatric illness is more common in individuals with epilepsy.
- 20–50% of individuals with epilepsy may suffer from depression.
- ~4x risk of suicide.
- Epileptic seizures themselves may be associated with mood disturbances and behavioural changes prior to, during and following a seizure.
- Temporal epilepsy may be associated with hallucinations and an increased risk of post-ictal psychosis.
- Delirium can occur following a seizure.
- Epilepsy may also be related to an increased risk of psychosis.

HIV	• Human immunodeficiency virus (HIV) has a broad-ranging impact on the body.
	• Advanced HIV infection can involve nervous tissue.
	• Acquired immunodeficiency syndrome (AIDS)-related **dementia** can occur, as well as **HIV encephalitis**. This has decreased following the introduction of effective HIV therapies.
	• Immunosuppression can allow opportunistic infections, which may have direct involvement with the brain parenchyma and present with psychiatric symptoms.
	• Adjustment disorder can occur following diagnosis.
	• Depression and anxiety are common in individuals diagnosed with HIV.

Sleep disorders[13–16]

Insomnia is a broad term relating to difficulty getting to or staying asleep, early waking or poor-quality sleep.

- **Short-term insomnia** – Sleep difficulties for <3 months
- **Long-term insomnia** – Sleep difficulties for 3 months or longer

Insomnia is common; ~1 in 3 individuals experience problems with sleep at least once a week.

Insomnia has a significant impact on an individual's quality of life and day-to-day functioning; it has also been linked to increased cardiovascular risks and is likely to impact many mental health conditions.

Aetiology

The causes of insomnia are wide-ranging; following are examples of common causes:

- Psychological stress.
- Mood disorders.
- Dementia and delirium – Often present with an altered sleep–wake cycle.
- Substance misuse.
- Prescribed medication and stimulants.
- Pain.
- Physical health conditions – Particularly conditions such as airway disease, heart failure, prostatism, musculoskeletal conditions.
- Episodic movement disorders – e.g., restless leg syndrome, periodic leg movements.

ASSESSMENT

- Full history of sleep symptoms – History of the sleep problem, frequency of problems, review of sleeping routines and environment, collateral history from those sharing a bed, impact on day-to-day life.

- Review of medical history.
- Medication review.
- Drug and alcohol history review.
- A sleep diary may be considered – Noting duration and quality of sleep and any problems experiences, triggers, times of meals and activities.
- Further medical investigations may be required.
- Referral to sleep specialists for video recording and polysomnography may be considered.

Management

Initial management recommendations:

- Address any comorbidities and triggers for poor sleep.
- Review sleep hygiene.

Short-term insomnia:

- Offer CBT for insomnia (CBT-I).
- Consider a short course of Z-drug if significant distress is observed.

Chronic insomnia:

- Offer CBT-I.
- Medication is not recommended for chronic insomnia.

SPECIFIC SLEEP DISORDERS

- Obstructive sleep apnoea – In obstructive sleep apnoea, the upper airway narrows or collapses during sleep, causing obstruction of breathing and apnoeic episodes.
- Restless leg syndrome – Individuals often experience unpleasant sensations in their legs accompanied by an urge to move them (this can ease the symptoms). Onset occurs in the evening and whilst awake but can make it difficult to sleep. Associated with Parkinson's, middle age, female sex, pregnancy and iron deficiency.
- Narcolepsy – Narcolepsy results in sudden episodes of sleep or excessive sleepiness during the day. Narcolepsy can be seen alongside **cataplexy** – sudden-onset loss of tone. These episodes occur despite a full night's sleep. Types of narcolepsy have been linked to **reduction in orexin levels**.
- Circadian rhythm disorders

  - Jet lag – Resulting from adjusting to a different time zone.
  - Shift work disorder – Resulting from shift workers having to adjust their sleeping patterns as a result of shift work.
  - Delayed sleep phase syndrome – Sleeping pattern is delayed or shifted to a later time, e.g., going to bed at 2:00 am and waking up in the afternoon.

- Parasomnias – Abnormal behaviour or activity during sleep.

  - Nightmares – Frightening dreams that are remembered after waking. Typically occur in rapid eye movement (REM) sleep.
  - Night terrors – Experience of terror often accompanied by screaming and autonomic activity; there is usually amnesia of the event. Occurs in early childhood (5–7 years old). Episodes occur in non-REM sleep.
  - Somnambulism – Sleep walking, most common in children (5–12 years old) but can persist into adulthood. Generally occurs in slow-wave sleep.
  - REM sleep disorder – Bodily movements occurring at night that often appear to be acting out a dream. Onset tends to occur in middle or old age. In older adults, movements can be associated with the onset of neurodegenerative disease such as Parkinson's disease or motor neurone disease.

Chronic fatigue syndrome[15,17]

Epidemiology

- Prevalence of 0.5% in the UK.
- More common in females than males.
- Typical onset 20–50 years old.

Aetiology

- The underlying cause of chronic fatigue syndrome is not clearly understood, and the impact of biological and psychological factors has been proposed.
- Biological factors – Viral infection (e.g., Lyme disease, hepatitis), immune or inflammatory activity, endocrine abnormalities.
- Psychological factors – Depression and anxiety disorders, personality traits, significant life stress, coping mechanisms, social factors.

Presentation

- Chronic fatigue syndrome can present with a broad range of symptoms across the body.
- Symptoms should be present for at least **3 months** prior to diagnosis.
- **Core symptoms:**

  - Severe fatigue which impacts on an individual's ability to engage in their day-to-day life.
  - "Post-exertional malaise" – Symptoms are exacerbated by activity and are out of proportion to the activity engaged in, with a prolonged recovery time.

- Altered sleeping patterns – Sleep is generally unrefreshing, and individuals feel exhausted upon waking.
- Cognitive symptoms – Poor concentration and memory, "**brain fog**" symptoms.

Management

- Initial assessment should include a whole-person assessment alongside relevant investigations to rule out underlying organic causes.
- Management should take a person-centred approach, acknowledging the impact of the condition on an individual's life and their own recovery goals.
- Awareness of the stigma that can be attached to individuals with chronic fatigue syndrome.
- Multidisciplinary approaches can be helpful, and treatment may include:
  - Medical review and symptom management.
  - Education around the diagnosis and management.
  - Treatment of any comorbid mood disorders or psychiatric conditions.
  - Psychological input.
  - Physiotherapeutic input – Establishing baseline functioning and supporting individuals in maintaining function. Graded exercise has been proposed but remains contentious.
  - Occupational and educational support.
  - Social worker involvement – May support with adaptations, caregiver assessments and support.

Emergency psychiatry

Self-harm and suicide

Epidemiology

Self-harm – UK Adult Psychiatric Morbidity Survey 2014[49]

- 7.3% of the population reported to have ever self-harmed.
- Females were more likely than males to have reported having ever self-harmed (8.9% of females and 5.7% of males).
- Self-harm is much more common in the younger population (aged under 34) and the group with the highest rate was females aged under 24 (25.7%).
- Individuals who have self-harmed have a lifetime risk of suicide of between 3–5%.

Thoughts of suicide – UK Adult Psychiatric Morbidity Survey 2014[49]

- 5.4% of individuals reported having suicidal thoughts in the past year and 20.6% reported also having these thoughts at an earlier time.

- Thoughts of suicide are more common in women (22.4%) than in men (18.7%).
- Younger individuals (<65 years) were more likely to report suicidal thoughts than those >65 years old.

Suicide attempts[49,63]

- 1 in 15 individuals has attempted to end their life at some point in time.
- Women (8%) are more likely to have attempted suicide than men (5.4%).
- Just over 50% of individuals sought help after attempting suicide.
- 1 in 100 individuals who are seen in hospital for a suicide attempt will end their life within a year, and 5 in 100 will do so within a decade.

Suicide[63,64]

- 5583 suicides were reported in England and Wales in 2021 (similar figures in previous years).
- Around 75% of individuals who die by suicide are male.
- 2021 Office of National Statistics (ONS) data shows that for women, individuals aged 45–49 years have the highest suicide rate, and for men, those aged 50–54 years have the highest suicide rate.
- 1 in 4 individuals who take their own life have accessed mental health services within the last year. 24% of these had recently been discharged from hospital.
- Individuals who have self-harmed have a lifetime risk of suicide of between 3–5%.

Suicide method – ONS 2021[64]

- Hanging, strangulation or suffocation is the most common method of suicide for both men and women (58.4% in 2021).
- Poisoning is the second most common method of suicide (20.5% in 2021). Other methods were much less frequent:

  - Jumping or lying in front of a moving object (3.8%).
  - Drowning (3.5%).
  - Sharp object (3.5%).
  - Falling (3.2%).
  - Other (7%).

Risks factors for suicide and suicidality

- Isolation – Living alone.
- Divorce – Greater risk factor for men than for women.
- Physical health problems particularly chronic pain.

- Comorbid mental health problems – Almost all mental health problems have been linked to suicide, most significantly depressive illness and drug and alcohol dependence, with 36–90% of individuals who completed suicide being diagnosed with depression, 43–54% being diagnosed with alcohol dependence, and 5–44% being diagnosed with personality disorder.
- Death of a loved one.
- Unemployment.
- Individuals on benefits – In 2014, 66.4% of individuals on employment support allowance reported having suicidal thoughts and 43.2% had made a suicide attempt at some point.
- Access to a means of suicide.
- Substance misuse.
- Social stressors.
- Occupation – doctors (2x risk), nurses (4x risk), farmers, veterinarians.
- Previous self-harm or suicide attempt – Particularly in older adults.

Risk assessment in self-harm and suicidality

- Risk assessments form an important part of all psychiatric assessments.
- Whilst looked at in isolation here, in practice, elements of a risk assessment can reflect an individual's entire psychiatric history.
- Friends and family members, alongside any witnesses, can provide important information, and information should always be sought from these individuals.
- Where an individual is accompanied by friends and family, it is important to also review them on their own, as there may be details they do not wish to disclose in front of others.

Important factors to explore:

- The events leading up to the act:

  - What has been going on in the life of the individual at the time leading up to the act?
  - Are there any recent triggers or stressors that might have precipitated the act?
  - How long had the individual been thinking about the act?
  - Had they done any research or planning, e.g., researching methods?
  - Had they made a will or put their affairs in order?
  - Had they written a suicide note?

- The event itself:

  - Was this an impulsive or in-the-moment event?
  - Had they made attempts not to be found?
  - Had they told anyone what they were going to do?

- What method did the individual use, and what was the outcome of this?
- What did they intend to happen?
- Had they been intoxicated or used substances at the time?

- Following the event:

  - How did they come to be seen in hospital?
  - How do they feel about what happened?
  - Do they have any current thoughts of self-harm or suicide?
  - Have any circumstances changed since this act?
  - Looking forward, what would they like to do now?
  - How do they see the future?

- Assessment of current psychiatric illness, e.g., depression, psychosis etc.
- Review of past psychiatric history, including previous self-harm.
- Physical health – Particularly thinking about chronic illness and pain.
- Social history – Including important friendships and relationships, accommodations, financial worries (e.g., debt), substance misuse.
- Safety planning – Forming a safe crisis plan helps you to understand the support structures for an individual, as well as their coping mechanism.

  - How might an individual identify that they are in crisis?
  - Are there any ongoing triggers?
  - Who does the individual live with?
  - Who might they be able to speak to if they felt that they were in crisis?
  - How might they seek help if they were in a crisis?

Support following an episode of self-harm or suicide attempt[67]

- Following an episode of self-harm or attempted suicide, individuals and their families should be involved in decision making about follow-up care.
- A safe discharge plan may involve:

  - Discharge home with support from a community team or their GP.
  - Discharge home with support from the crisis/home treatment team.
  - Admission to a mental health hospital, either informally or under the mental health act, for a period of assessment and risk management.

- Care should be taken to consider any comorbid psychiatric conditions and any support required.
- Individuals who have self-harmed should be offered the opportunity to engage in psychological support around self-harm.
- Individuals should be given a clear care plan which has been formulated jointly with them.
- Individuals should be given information on who to seek help from in the event of a crisis.

Other psychiatric emergencies

The following chart is taken from the first book in this series, "Revision Guide for MRCPsych Paper A".[76]

All emergencies	In all emergencies, in line with national guidelines, staff should ensure their own safety prior to assessing the patient. They should call for help and assess the patient using approaches taught in basic and intermediate life support courses, in which all staff should have training. An ambulance should be called immediately if there are any physical health concerns. Trust guidelines should be followed where available.
Dystonic reaction	An acute dystonic reaction is characterised by involuntary contractions of muscles of the extremities, face, neck, abdomen, pelvis, or larynx, in either sustained or intermittent patterns, that lead to abnormal movements or postures. The aetiology of an acute dystonic reaction is thought to be due to neurotransmitter imbalance in the basal ganglia. A number of medications can be used in the treatment of dystonic reactions, including benztropine, diphenhydramine, benzodiazepines and trihexyphenidyl. Clinicians should stop the responsible medication, and supportive measures in hospital are advised.
Oculogyric crisis	An oculogyric crisis occurs when there is a spasm of the extraocular muscles leading to tonic, usually upward deviation of the eye. Each spasm can last from seconds to several hours. An oculogyric crisis is associated with the use of medications including antidepressants, antipsychotics and antiemetics (metoclopramide is strongly associated with precipitating this side effect in females). A number of medications can be used in the treatment of an oculogyric crisis, including benztropine, diphenhydramine, benzodiazepines and trihexyphenidyl. Clinicians should stop the responsible medication and seek further medical support as necessary.
Neuroleptic malignant syndrome and serotonin syndrome	Early recognition is crucial. Treatment involves stopping the responsible agent and transferring the patient to a physical health hospital. Supportive treatment is the main recommendation, but benzodiazepines may be used. Intubation and intensive care support with specialist drugs may be required.
Hanging	If a patient is found hanging, staff should call for help and ensure that a ligature cutter is used to release the ligature with controlled c-spine stabilisation and support of the head and neck. Ward staff should have training in cutting a ligature and should avoid the knot. An individual cannot do this safely without support from colleagues. Further medical assistance should follow in line with life support guidance and in relation to the injuries sustained.

Deliberate self-harm	Management of a deliberate self-harming incident is dependent on the method of self-harm, any object used to cause injury and the degree of injury caused. Where possible, remove the object used to cause injury and treat any acute medical problems. Ensure that smaller injuries are not neglected and consider reviewing leave and other safety plans in place. Conduct risk assessment to ensure patient safety and remove further objects that may be with the patient that could cause harm to themselves or others.
Medication overdose	If a patient has experienced a medication overdose, it is important to ensure they no longer have access to the medication source or stockpile. Depending on the medication or combination of medications that have been taken, a physical health review in the accident and emergency department will be required, and doubt exists, further discussion with an acute hospital physician is suggested.
	Certain medications will have specific management treatments, for example N-acetylcysteine (NAC) in paracetamol overdose, and specialist advice should be sought, with toxicology resources such as TOXBASE referred to for guidance. Certain medications are particularly dangerous in overdose, for example the TCAs amitriptyline, dosulepin and doxepin; these should be avoided in patients who are at a high risk of overdose.
Violent incidents	All violent incidents should be managed in 3 stages:
	Acutely, any physical injuries should be attended to, safety prioritised and de-escalation used where possible, with physical restraint, rapid tranquilisation and seclusion used as a last resort.
	The incident should be documented and a safety incident form submitted using the online adverse incident reporting system.
	A safety huddle or space for reflection should be used within the team to learn from the event.

Emergency aspects of the Mental Health Act[75]

The Mental Health Act sets out laws around the assessment and management of those with mental health problems.

The Mental Health Code of Practice provides information on understanding and interpreting the mental health act and can be found online for free.

Relevant to emergency psychiatry are the laws around detention and compulsory care for individuals under the Mental Health Act.

An individual can only be detained under the mental health act if it is felt that:

- They are suffering from a mental health condition of a nature or degree that warrants detention.
- Detention is required in the interests of the individual's health and safety or the safety of others.

- Admission to hospital is required.
- Admission to hospital cannot be done voluntarily (either because the individual lacks capacity or is not in agreement to this).

Following is a description of relevant sections.

Section 135

Police are able to obtain a warrant from the local magistrate in order to **access someone's home to facilitate an assessment under the mental health act**.

This enables police to detain someone in a place of safety for a period of **24 hours**, which can be further extended by 12 hours in specific circumstances.

Section 136

Police are able to detain someone who is **in a public space in order to bring them to a place of safety** to enable an assessment by mental health professionals.

This enables police to detain someone in a place of safety for a period of **24 hours**, which can be further extended by 12 hours in specific circumstances.

During this time an individual must be assessed by a minimum of an approved mental health practitioner (**AMHP**) and ideally a Section 12-approved doctor.

Section 5(2)

An application made by a single doctor detaining an individual for a period of up to **72 hours** for their safety and further assessment.

Section 5(4)

An application made by a single nurse to detain an individual for a period of up to **6 hours**. This is to allow for further assessment by a doctor. A Section 5(4) event will come to an end following an assessment by a doctor, so a decision around the appropriateness of further detention is required.

Section 2

Detention under Section 2 of the mental health act requires an assessment take place including:

- A doctor from the assessing team – Ideally Section 12-approved.
- An independent doctor – They must not work within the same team as the first doctor.
- An **AMHP**.

The purpose of detention under Section 2 of the mental health act is to allow for a **period of assessment** of an individual and their mental health needs.

Individuals detained under Section 2 of the mental health act can be detained for a **maximum period of 28 days**.

Detention under Section 2 **cannot be extended**, and further detention under the mental health act requires further assessment.

Individuals **can be treated against their will** under Section 2 of the mental health act.

Individuals **have the right to appeal** their detention under Section 2 of the mental health act.

Section 3

Detention under Section 3 of the mental health act requires an assessment take place including:

- A doctor from the assessing team – Ideally Section 12-approved.
- An independent doctor – They must not work within the same team as the first doctor.
- An **AMHP**.

The purpose of detention under Section 3 of the mental health act is **to allow for treatment of a mental illness. An appropriate treatment plan must be** considered and **made available** as part of this assessment.

Individuals detained under Section 3 of the mental health act can be detained for a **period of 6 months**.

Detention under Section 3 **can be further extended if required.**

Individuals **can be treated against their will** under Section 3 of the mental health act.

Individuals **have the right to appeal** their detention under Section 3 of the mental health act.

Section 4

Section 4 is an **emergency section used when only 1 doctor and an AMHP are available.**

Individuals can be detained for a maximum period of **72 hours** by Section 4.

Following assessment by an additional independent doctor, a **Section 4 detainment can be converted into a Section 2 detainment.**

This section is not commonly used in practice.

Psychosexual disorders[14,68]

- Sexual disorders are often a complex mix of organic, psychological and sometimes iatrogenic factors.

- Full assessment and management are likely to follow an MDT approach, often drawing across specialisms including endocrinology and urology.
- Psychiatrists and psychologists may be involved in supporting this MDT.

Non-organic sexual dysfunction[69]

The DSM and ICD include classifications of non-organic sexual dysfunction disorders. These can be grouped into the follow 4 categories:

- **Sex drive** – Loss of or lack of sexual desire, "excessive sexual drive," alongside aversion to or the lack of sexual enjoyment.
- **Arousal** – "failure of genital response" or erectile disorder – relates to erectile dysfunction in men or lack of arousal and vaginal dryness/lack of lubrication in women.
- **Orgasmic dysfunction** – Where orgasm either does not occur (anorgasmia) or is delayed or premature.
- **Pain disorders** – Genitopelvic pain/penetration disorder or non-organic vaginismus (spasming of pelvic floor often causing pain or difficult in penetration), dyspareunia, painful ejaculations.

Psychiatrists should be particularly aware of the following psychoactive drugs and their impact on sexual dysfunction – Antidepressants, lithium, antipsychotics, benzodiazepines, antihistamines, Parkinson's medication.

- 40–70% of people on antipsychotics experience sexual dysfunction.
- 50% of individuals on SSRIs experience change in sexual function.[70]

Management

Management is likely to vary dependent on individual cases:

- Couples are generally treated together.
- Full history of the problem should be assessed, along with physical examination and blood tests including sex hormones such as prolactin, diabetic monitoring and other laboratory tests.
- Education of the anatomy, physiology and psychology surrounding sex.
- Counselling/support around communications.
- Medication may be involved in management.

  - Sildenafil is commonly used in erectile dysfunction.
  - SSRIs are sometimes used in premature ejaculation.
  - Topical lubricants or analgesics are sometimes used in pain disorders and disorders of arousal for women.
  - "Insertion trainers" are sometimes used in vaginismus.
  - Sex-hormone replacement – Either topical or systemic in individuals with low levels.

Paraphilias[71]

Paraphilias disorders of sexual preference, they reflect individual sexual desires that are seen as either not the norm or harmful to others or oneself.

ICD-10 Classifies the following paraphilias:

- Fetishism – Sexual arousal experienced from non-living objects or from parts of the body that are not directly sexual, e.g., rubber or shoes.
- Fetishistic transvestism – Deriving sexual pleasure from the wearing of clothes from the opposite gender. Importantly, the individual does not desire to live as the opposite gender.
- Exhibitionism – Sexual pleasure derived from being observed, particularly from exposing genitalia in public. ICD-10 states that this is without the desire for initiating sexual relations.
- Voyeurism – Sexual pleasure gained from watching others without their knowledge.
- Paedophilia – Sexual preference for children.
- Sadomasochism – Pleasure derived from pain, humiliation and bondage. A sadist gains pleasure in giving this stimulation and a masochist gains pleasure in receiving this.
- Multiple or other.

Gender incongruence, including transsexualism and transvestism

Overview[14,74]

- Prevalence of gender incongruence is estimated at ~0.5–1%.
- ICD-10 had previously used the categories of gender identity disorder and transsexualism; these have been replaced by gender incongruence.
- Psychiatrists' roles in supporting individuals with gender incongruence is evolving, as is the classification system.
- Gender incongruence tends to be managed in specialist clinics involving an MDT of psychiatrists, psychotherapists, endocrinologists and other medical professionals.
- Its likely that our approaches to this topic will change significantly over coming years.
- Gender incongruence receives significant stigma and is currently a topic of widespread media debate, which is likely to impact in individual's mental health and wellbeing.
- Individuals with gender incongruence often have significant comorbid mental health difficulties, particularly anxiety and depression.

ICD-10 categories[72]

- Transsexualism – Described as the desire to live as a member of the opposite sex, individuals will experience an intense dysphoria (distress and discomfort) towards the sex that they were assigned at birth.

- Dual-role transvestism – Described as an individual who wishes to wear the clothes of the opposite sex and "to enjoy the temporary experience of membership of the opposite sex" but does not wish to live as the opposite sex.
- Gender identity disorder of childhood – Described as occurring in early childhood, where an individual experiences intense distress around the sex they were assigned at birth and a desire to live as the opposite sex. The description includes "a persistent preoccupation with the dress and activities of the opposite sex and repudiation of the individual's own sex."

ICD-11[73]

- There is a single category of gender incongruence, which is split between adolescence/adulthood and childhood.
- Gender incongruence is placed alongside "Conditions Related to Sexual Health."
- Definition:

"Gender incongruence is characterised by a marked and persistent incongruence between an individual's experienced gender and the assigned sex."

References

1. Public mental health: Evidence, practice and commissioning. *Royal College of Psychiatrists*, May 2019, www.rsph.org.uk/static/uploaded/b215d040-2753-410e-a39eb30ad3c8b708.pdf
2. Paul Harrison, Philip Cowen, Tom Burns, Mina Fazel. Chapter 9. Depression. In *Shorter Oxford textbook of psychiatry*, 7th edition. Oxford University Press, 2017.
3. NICE clinical knowledge summaries. *Depression*, September 2022, https://cks.nice.org.uk/topics/depression/
4. ICD10. *WHO, Depression F32*, https://icd.who.int/browse10/2019/en#/F32
5. Depression in adults: Treatment and management. *NICE Guidelines 222*, June 2022, www.nice.org.uk/guidance/ng222/chapter/Recommendations
6. David Taylor, Thomas Barns, Allan Young. Chapter 3. Depression and anxiety. In *Maudsley prescribing guidelines in psychiatry*, 14th edition. John Wiley, 2021.
7. Sarah Stringer, Laurence Church, Susan Davison, Maurice Lipsedge. Chapter 7. Affective disorders. In *Psychiatry P.R.N. Principles reality next steps*. Oxford University Press, 2009
8. Adam Feather, David Randall, Mona Waterhouse. Chapter 21. Neurological disease. In *Kumar and Clark's clinical medicine*, 7th edition. Elsevier Health Sciences, 2009.
9. Sarah Stringer, Laurence Church, Susan Davison, Maurice Lipsedge. Chapter 11. Organic psychiatry. In *Psychiatry P.R.N. Principles reality next steps*. Oxford University Press, 2009.
10. Paul Harrison, Philip Cowen, Tom Burns, Mina Fazel. Chapter 14. Dementia, delirium and other neuropsychiatric disorders. In *Shorter Oxford textbook of psychiatry*, 7th edition. Oxford University Press, 2017.
11. Joseph Jankovic, Mark Hallett, Michael S. Okun, Cynthia Comella, Stanley Fahn, Jennifer Goldman. Chapter 13. In *Principles and practice of movement disorders*. Elsevier, 2021.

12. Adam Feather, David Randall, Mona Waterhouse. Chapter 7. Liver, biliary tract and pancreatic disease neurological disease. In *Kumar and Clark's clinical medicine*, 7th edition. Elsevier.

13. Nancy J. Newman, Joseph Jankovic, John C. Mazziotta. *Bradley and Daroff's neurology in clinical practice*, 8th edition. Elsevier, 2021.

14. Paul Harrison, Philip Cowen, Tom Burns, Mina Fazel. Chapter 13. Eating, sleep and sexual disorders. In *Shorter Oxford textbook of psychiatry*, 7th edition. Oxford University Press, 2017.

15. Adam Feather, David Randall, Mona Waterhouse. Chapter 22. Psychological medicine. In *Kumar and Clark's clinical medicine*, 7th edition. Elsevier, 2009.

16. NICE CKS Insomnia, May 2022, https://cks.nice.org.uk/topics/insomnia/

17. NICE Guidelines 206. *Chronic Fatigue Syndrome*, October 2021 (Myalgic encephalomyelitis (or encephalopathy)/chronic fatigue syndrome: Diagnosis and management). Scenario: Management | Management | Tiredness/fatigue in adults | CKS | NICE.

18. Paul Harrison, Philip Cowen, Tom Burns, Mina Fazel. Chapter 10. Bipolar disorder. In *Shorter Oxford textbook of psychiatry*, 7th edition. Oxford University Press.

19. Bipolar Disorder. *NICE CKS*, October 2022, https://cks.nice.org.uk/topics/bipolar-disorder/

20. Bipolar disorder: Assessment and management. *Nice Guidance CG185*, February 2020, www.nice.org.uk/guidance/cg185

21. ICD 10 Mood [Affective] disorders (F30-F39). *WHO*, https://icd.who.int/browse10/2019/en#/F30-F39

22. ICD 11 Bipolar or related disorders. *WHO*, https://icd.who.int/browse11/l-m/en#/http%3a%2f%2fid.who.int%2ficd%2fentity%2f613065957

23. David Taylor, Thomas Barns, Allan Young. Chapter 2. Bipolar disorder. In *Maudsley prescribing guidelines in psychiatry*, 14th edition. Elsevier.

24. Sarah Stringer, Laurence Church, Susan Davison, Maurice Lipsedge. Chapter 9. Schizophrenia. In *Psychiatry P.R.N. Principles reality next steps*. Oxford University Press, 2009.

25. NICE CKS psychosis and schizophrenia, September 2021. https://cks.nice.org.uk/topics/psychosis-schizophrenia/

26. Psychosis and schizophrenia in adults: Prevention and management. *NICE Guidelines 178*, February 2014. www.nice.org.uk/guidance/cg178

27. Paul Harrison, Philip Cowen, Tom Burns, Mina Fazel. Chapter 11. Schizophrenia. In *Shorter Oxford textbook of psychiatry*, 7th edition. Oxford University Press.

28. Schizophrenia, schizotypal and delusional disorders, (F20-F29), *ICD10*. WHO, https://icd.who.int/browse10/2019/en#/F20-F29

29. David Taylor, Thomas Barns, Allan Young. Chapter 1. Schizophrenia and related psychosis. In *Maudsley prescribing guidelines in psychiatry*, 14th edition. John Wiley.

30. Schizoaffective disorder. *BMJ Best Practice*. https://bestpractice.bmj.com/topics/en-gb/1199?q=Schizoaffective%20disorder&c=suggested

31. Paul Harrison, Philip Cowen, Tom Burns, Mina Fazel. Chapter 12. Paranoid symptoms and syndromes. In *Shorter Oxford textbook of psychiatry*, 7th edition. Oxford University Press.

32. Paul Harrison, Philip Cowen, Tom Burns, Mina Fazel. Chapter 22. Psychiatric aspects of medical procedures and conditions In *Shorter Oxford textbook of psychiatry*, 7th edition. Oxford University Press.

33. Adam Feather, David Randall, Mona Waterhouse. Chapter 4. Infection and infectious diseases. In *Kumar and Clark's clinical medicine*, 7th edition. Elsevier.

34. Common mental health disorders: Full guideline. *NICE Guidelines 123*, May 2011. www.nice.org.uk/guidance/cg123/evidence/full-guideline-181771741

35. Sarah Stringer, Laurence Church, Susan Davison, Maurice Lipsedge. Chapter 13. Anxiety, obsessions, and reactions to stress. In *Psychiatry P.R.N. Principles reality next steps*. Oxford University Press, 2009.

36. Paul Harrison, Philip Cowen, Tom Burns, Mina Fazel. Chapter 8. Anxiety and Obsessive-compulsive disorders. In *Shorter Oxford textbook of psychiatry*, 7th edition. Oxford University Press.

37. Neurotic, stress-related and somatoform disorders. *ICD 10 WHO*, https://icd.who.int/browse10/2019/en#/F40-F48

38. Generalised anxiety disorder and panic disorder in adults: Management. *NICE Guidelines 113*, June 2020. www.nice.org.uk/guidance/cg113

39. Generalised Anxiety disorder. *NICE CKS*. https://cks.nice.org.uk/topics/generalized-anxiety-disorder/

40. Paul Harrison, Philip Cowen, Tom Burns, Mina Fazel. Chapter 7. Reactions to stress. In *Shorter Oxford textbook of psychiatry*, 7th edition. Oxford University Press.

41. Post traumatic stress disorder. *NICE CKS*, August 2022. https://cks.nice.org.uk/topics/post-traumatic-stress-disorder/

42. Post traumatic stress disorder. *NICE Guidelines 116*, December 2018, www.nice.org.uk/guidance/ng116

43. Obsessive compulsive disorder. *NICE CKS*, June 2018, https://cks.nice.org.uk/topics/obsessive-compulsive-disorder/

44. Obsessive compulsive disorder and body dysmorphic disorder: Treatment. *NICE Guidelines*, 31 November 2005, www.nice.org.uk/guidance/cg31

45. Sarah Stringer, Laurence Church, Susan Davison, Maurice Lipsedge. Chapter 14. Medically unexplained symptoms. In *Psychiatry P.R.N. Principles reality next steps*. Oxford University Press, 2009.

46. Sarah Stringer, Laurence Church, Susan Davison, Maurice Lipsedge. Chapter 20. Personality disorders. In *Psychiatry P.R.N. Principles reality next steps*. Oxford University Press, 2009.

47. Paul Harrison, Philip Cowen, Tom Burns, Mina Fazel. Chapter 15. Dementia, personality and personality disorders. In *Shorter Oxford textbook of psychiatry*, 7th edition. Oxford University Press.

48. Mark F. Lenzenweger. Epidemiology of personality disorders. *Psychiatric Clinics of North America*, 31(3), 95–403.

49. Adult psychiatric morbidity survey: Survey of mental health and wellbeing, England, 2014, 29 Sep 2016, https://digital.nhs.uk/data-and-information/publications/statistical/adult-psychiatric-morbidity-survey/adult-psychiatric-morbidity-survey-survey-of-mental-health-and-wellbeing-england-2014

50. ICD 10 WHO Disorders of adult personality and behaviour (F60-F69), https://icd.who.int/browse10/2019/en#/F60-F69

51. ICD 11, WHO, 6D10 personality disorders, https://icd.who.int/browse11/l-m/en#/http://id.who.int/icd/entity/941859884

52. Borderline personality disorder: Recognition and management. *NICE Guidelines 78*, January 2009, www.nice.org.uk/guidance/cg78/chapter/1-Guidance

53. Sarah Stringer, Laurence Church, Susan Davison, Maurice Lipsedge, Chapter 17. Problems following childbirth. In *Psychiatry P.R.N. Principles reality next steps*. Oxford University Press, 2009.

54. Depression – Antenatal and post natal. *NICE CKS*, April 2022. https://cks.nice.org.uk/topics/depression-antenatal-postnatal/

55. Paul Harrison, Philip Cowen, Tom Burns, Mina Fazel. Chapter 25. Drugs and other physical treatments. In *Shorter Oxford textbook of psychiatry*, 7th edition. Oxford University Press.

56. Antenatal and postnatal mental health: Clinical management and service guidance. *NICE Guidelines 192*, December 2014, www.nice.org.uk/guidance/cg192/resources/antenatal-and-postnatal-mental-health-clinical-management-and-service-guidance-pdf-35109869806789

57. David Taylor, Thomas Barns, Allan Young. Chapter 7. Pregnancy and breast feeding. In *Maudsley prescribing guidelines in psychiatry*, 14th edition. Elsevier.

58. Runjhun Bhatia, Carolyn Bevan, Elizabeth E. Neurologic disorders in pregnancy. Gerard. In *Gabbe's obstetrics: Normal and problem pregnancies*, 8th edition. Elsevier.

59. Kenneth E. Freedland, Robert M. Carney, Eric J. Lenze, Michael W. Rich. Psychiatric and psychosocial aspects of cardiovascular disease. In *Braunwald's heart disease: A textbook of cardiovascular medicine*, 12th edition. Elsevier.

60. David Taylor, Thomas Barns, Allan Young. ECG changes – QT prolongation. In *Maudsley prescribing guidelines in psychiatry*, 14th edition. Elsevier.

61. Adam Feather, David Randall, Mona Waterhouse. Diabetes mellitus. In *Kumar and Clark's clinical medicine*, 10th edition. London: Richard I.G. Holt

62. David Taylor, Thomas Barns, Allan Young. Chapter 8. Hepatic and renal impairment. In *Maudsley prescribing guidelines in psychiatry*, 14th edition. Elsevier.

63. Suicide Fact Sheet. South West London and St Georges NHS trust, www.swl-stg.nhs.uk/documents/related-documents/news-and-events/reporting-guidelines/reporting-suicides/105-suicide-factsheet/file

64. Suicides in England and Wales: 2021 registrations. *Office for National Statistics*, September 2022, www.ons.gov.uk/peoplepopulationandcommunity/birthsdeathsandmarriages/deaths/bulletins/suicidesintheunitedkingdom/2021r egistrations

65. Paul Harrison, Philip Cowen, Tom Burns, Mina Fazel. Chapter 21. Suicide and deliberate self-harm. In *Shorter Oxford textbook of psychiatry*, 7th edition. Oxford University Press.

66. Sarah Stringer, Laurence Church, Susan Davison, Maurice Lipsedge. Chapter 8. Suicide and self-harm. In *Psychiatry P.R.N. Principles reality next steps*. Oxford University Press, 2009.

67. Self-harm: assessment, management and preventing recurrence. *Nice Guidelines 225*, September 2022, www.nice.org.uk/guidance/ng225/chapter/Recommendations#interventions-for-self-harm

68. Sarah Stringer, Laurence Church, Susan Davison, Maurice Lipsedge. Chapter 16. Psychosexual disorders. In *Psychiatry P.R.N. Principles reality next steps*. Oxford University Press, 2009.

69. Sexual dysfunction not caused by organic disorder. *ICD10, WHO*, https://icd.who.int/browse10/2019/en#/F52

70. MacDonald SM, Burnett AL. Physiology of erection and pathophysiology of erectile dysfunction. *Urologic Clinics of North America*, 48(4), 513–525. doi: 10.1016/j.ucl.2021.06.009. PMID: 34602172.

71. Disorders of sexual preference. *ICD10, WHO*, https://icd.who.int/browse10/2019/en#/F65

72. Gender identity disorder. *ICD10, WHO*, https://icd.who.int/browse10/2019/en#/F64

73. Gender Incongruence. *ICD 11, WHO*, https://icd.who.int/browse11/l-m/en#/http://id.who.int/icd/entity/411470068

74. Managing patients with gender incongruence. *BMA*, www.bma.org.uk/advice-and-support/gp-practices/gp-service-provision/managing-patients-with-gender-dysphoria

75. The mental health act 1983: Code of practice. *Department of Health*. https://assets.publishing.service.gov.uk/government/uploads/system/uploads/attachment_data/file/435512/MHA_Code_of_Practice.PDF

76. Elizabeth Templeton, Richard William Kerslake, Lisanne Stock. *Revision guide for MRCPsych paper A*, 1st edition. Elsevier.

4 Old age psychiatry

Richard William Kerslake

Demographic population changes in the UK and worldwide

Population demographics across the world are changing with respect to older people who require support for mental illness[1]. In the UK, the proportion of older people is expected to increase, with the number of people aged over 75 expected to double by 2046 (see Table 4.1).

Table 4.1 Changing demographic of the UK population[2]

	2016	2026	2036	2046
UK total population (millions)	65.6	69.2	71.8	73.9
Proportion aged 65+	18.0%	20.5%	23.9%	24.7%
Proportion aged 75+	8.1%	10.2%	12.1%	14.5%

The Social Care Institute for Excellence estimated that:

- 40% of older people attending general practice clinics have a mental health problem.
- 50% of older people in general hospitals have a mental health problem.
- 60% of those in care homes have a mental health problem.

The complexity of mental health challenges in older adults is also thought to be greater than that of the working-age population, with:

- Depression affecting 22% of men and 26% of women aged over 65, and 40% of older people in care homes[3].
- Anxiety affecting 5% of older adults[4].
- The prevalence of dementia amongst older people in the UK is expected to rise in 2040 by 80% to 1.59 million people[5].

The Alzheimer's Society reported that in the UK in 2019:

- The prevalence of dementia amongst older people was estimated to be 7.1%, a total of almost 885,000 people.

DOI: 10.4324/9781003376163-4

- Of these, 14.4% had mild dementia, 27.8% had moderate dementia, and 57.8% had severe dementia.
- By 2040, the number of people with severe dementia is expected to rise the most, by 109%, followed by mild dementia by 55% and moderate dementia by 33%.
- The total costs of supporting older people with dementia in the UK in 2019 was calculated as £34.7 billion and is expected to rise to £94.1 billion by 2040.

Worldwide, more than 46 million people were estimated to be living with dementia in 2015, and this figure is expected to rise to 131.5 million in 2050[6]. 60% of these individuals live in low- and middle-income economies. The global cost of dementia was estimated as $1.3 trillion in 2019. However, in the USA and Europe, the incidence has decreased by 25% over the past 20 years, implying that dementia is preventable[7].

District service provision, need for specialisation, principles of service provision, multidisciplinary working with reference to needs of an older population, relationships with and provision by social services and voluntary bodies, liaison with geriatricians and attention to the needs of carers

Supporting the mental health needs of older people requires a range of services across primary, secondary and tertiary care, in addition to adult social care and voluntary care sector organisations (VCSOs). The Community Mental Health Framework recognises that effective care for older adults requires all these organisations to work collaboratively[8]. Figure 4.1 demonstrates the aim of maintaining these individuals at the centre of their communities, using services as necessary.

An individual might engage with self-help or self-care to support their mental health.

Mental health support can be provided within a person's **personal community** by friends and family, neighbours, at work and through online and social media activities.

Wider, non-specific **community** resources, such as libraries, community centres, local events, faith groups, etc. also provide support to maintain a person's mental wellbeing.

Community-based health and social care is also available in the form of Improving Access to Psychological Therapies organisations, employment and housing support teams, general practice, VCSOs and carer support organisations.

Acute mental health care may be available where the previous layers of support have not been sufficient to maintain a person's mental health. This includes community mental health teams, crisis teams, mental health liaison teams and older persons' psychiatric inpatient units.

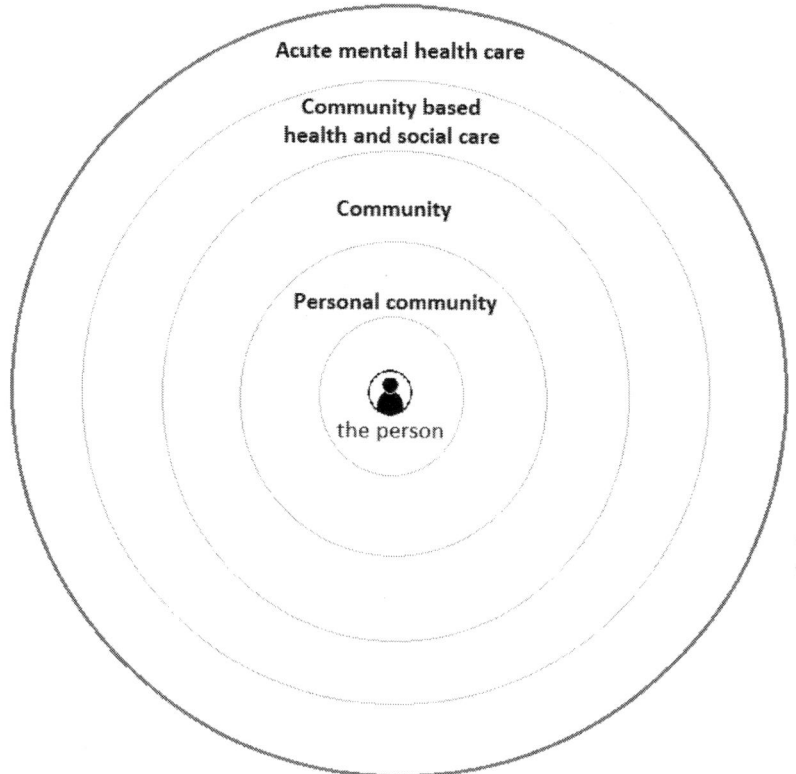

Figure 4.1 Integrated model of community mental health support

The description for old age psychiatry services in the UK[9] explains that access to older persons' mental health services should not be defined by age alone, and has developed needs-based criteria:

1. People of any age with a primary dementia.
2. People with a mental disorder and physical illness or frailty that contributes to, or complicates, the management of their mental illness (may include people <65 years).
3. People with psychological or social difficulties related to the ageing process, or end-of-life issues, or who feel their needs may be best met by a service for older people (normally includes people >70 years).

Older adults experience mental illness in a range of domains including affective, psychotic, cognitive, behavioural, personality, substance misuse and social disorders. The complexity in older adults requires specialist support from a range of disciplines practicing cohesively. The gold standard model of service delivery is through **multidisciplinary treatment teams (MDT)**[11],

Table 4.2 Key documents relevant to services for older adults

2001 – The National Service Framework for Older People	Quality standards for health and social care include: • *Helping older people to stay as healthy, active and independent as possible, for as long as possible.* • *Ensuring that older people are treated with respect.* • *Preventing unnecessary hospital admission and supporting early discharge.* • *Reducing long-term illness by providing specialist care.* • *Promoting healthy lifestyles and independence for those of older age.*
2005 – Everybody's Business[10]	This report made explicit that support for mental health in older people requires a coordinated approach for physical and mental health from both mainstream and specialist services, alongside health and social care networks.
2010 – The Equalities Act	This established a legal requirement to promote age equity in mental health delivery. This led to criticism of commissioning 'ageless' services as not valuing age-appropriateness and being a form of indirect discrimination.
2011 – No Health Without Mental Health	A cross-government strategy promoting mental health for people of all ages, with an expectation that services be age appropriate and non-discriminatory.
Joint Commissioning Panel for Older People's Mental Health	10 key points for mental health commissioning: *1. Older people will form a larger proportion of the population.* *2. Older people's mental health services in particular benefit from an integrated approach with social care services.* *3. Older people's mental health service providers need to work closely with primary care and community services.* *4. Services must be commissioned on the basis of need and not age alone.* *5. Older people's mental health services must address the needs of people with functional illnesses such as depression and psychosis, as well as dementia.* *6. Older people often have a combination of mental and physical health problems.* *7. Older people's mental health services must be disciplinary.* *8. Older people with mental health needs should have access to community crisis or home treatment services.* *9. Older people with mental health needs respond well to psychological input.* *10. Older people should have dedicated liaison services in acute hospitals.*

where the skills are specific to older people due to changes in physiology, frailty, social role and support needs. A typical MDT will involve:

Table 4.3 Members of the MDT

Nurses	Specialist skills in psychiatric and physical health care, care plan approach (CPA), community assessment and treatment, non-pharmacological interventions, understanding of Mental Health and Mental Capacity Act and clinical leadership.
Support workers	Non-pharmacological interventions, social support connections, physical health care and emotional and practical support.
Occupational therapists	Specialist assessment of mental health and physical needs, CPA coordination, discharge planning, non-pharmacological intervention, team supervision.
Psychologists	Specialist skills in talking therapies with a focus on the needs of older people and their carers, neuropsychiatric assessment with understanding of cognitive disorders, clinical assessment, formulation and team leadership.
Doctors	Specialist psychiatric knowledge, understanding of physiology and pharmacodynamics of older persons, mental health assessments and interventions and Mental Health and Mental Capacity Act considerations.

Administrators, dieticians, speech and language therapists and physiotherapists also provide invaluable support to teams where they are available.

Informal carers, usually relatives, are central to supporting the majority of older people with mental illness.

- 1 in 10 people in the UK provide unpaid care.
- 44% (£11.6 billion) of the total cost of dementia in the UK is from the work of unpaid carers[12].
- 55% of informal carers report they have suffered from depression as a result of their caring role[13], and carer strain is a recognised precipitant for an older person moving into a long-term care placement.

Specialist aspects of assessment of mental health in older people

Older people's mental health services should be provided to[14]:

- People of any age where dementia is the primary diagnosis.
- People with a mental disorder, where their physical illness or frailty complicates the management of their mental illness.
- People with psychological or social difficulties related to ageing or end-of-life matters.

Assessment of mental disorders in older adults must consider:

- Mood disorders: depression, anxiety and mania

- Psychosis: which may present as a primary or late-onset schizophrenia or paraphrenia, or may be a neuropsychiatric feature of underlying cognitive impairment.
- The role of psychological and neurocognitive assessment.
- Cognitive disorders: assessment of primary dementias, or dementias secondary to other conditions, including the role of diagnostic neuroimaging.
- Physical health factors that can mimic or influence mental illness. Presentation, diagnosis and treatment may be complicated by organic pathology; for example, depression may be the first symptom of undiagnosed dementia, and mood changes may be secondary to a cerebral event or small vessel disease. Physical health factors specific to ageing must also be considered in the support and medical management of older people.
- Substance misuse, social factors and personality disorders continue to have relevance in old age, but their impact can be unique in this population.
- Assessment of functional abilities and carer involvement are central to optimising quality of life and support for older people.
- The role of relevant legal frameworks, including the Mental Capacity Act (MCA), Mental Health Act (MHA) and Deprivation of Liberty Safeguards (DOLS).

Psychological aspects of physical disease; particular emphasis on possible psychiatric sequelae of Parkinson's disease, cerebrovascular disease, sensory impairment. Emotional reaction to illness and to chronic ill health. Secondary and reversible dementias

Parkinson's disease (PD)

Anxiety affects up to 55% of those diagnosed and depression affects up to 56%. Not all of this can be attributed to the neurobiology of the disorder, recognising the psychosocial impact of the diagnosis.

Psychosis is also common[15], with *visual hallucinations* being commonly reported, typically of well-formed persons, animals or objects, experienced with insight, and often as a result of Lewy body pathology.

Delusions are also reported, often erotomaniac, jealous and persecutory in nature, and tend to be due to dopamine agonist therapy used in the treatment of PD.

Impulse control disorders, including pathological gambling, hypersexuality, binge eating and compulsive buying, are also recognised as being related to dopamine agonist therapy[16].

Rapid eye movement (REM) behavioural sleep disturbance affects 47% of patients and negatively impacts interpersonal relationships and health-related quality of life[17].

Cerebrovascular disease

Cognitive symptoms are common, including impaired memory, concentration and speed of information processing.

Emotional consequences of stroke include depression (30%), anxiety (30%) and emotional lability (10–20%). These may be due to insults to the limbic system, or as a psychosocial consequence of the physical and cognitive effects of the disease.

The concept of *vascular depression* is recognised as a geriatric depressive syndrome influenced by cerebrovascular disease.

Behavioural changes, depending on the brain region affected by cerebrovascular disease, may include aggression, disinhibition, impulsivity and distractibility.

30–40% of people experience *delirium* in the week after a stroke.

Sensory impairment

Charles Bonnet Syndrome is the experience of complex visual hallucinations, with insight usually retained, as a consequence of significant visual impairment and not due to mental disorder. Vision loss in the form of central visual acuity, usually due to macular degeneration.

Hearing impairment in mid-life has a relative risk for dementia of 1.9, with the highest population-attributable fraction of any mid-life risk factor[18]. Those who wear hearing aids are not affected by cognitive decline.

Chronic ill health

As life expectancy increases, the risk of health comorbidity also increases, and with it the emotional cost of treatment and surveillance. For example, the prevalence of an affective disorder amongst patients admitted with diabetes or rheumatoid arthritis is 20–25%[19].

Diagnosis of depression is also complicated by physical illness, which can equally affect appetite, sleep and energy levels.

Medical conditions in the elderly are often life-limiting and can affect an individual's capacity to view the future with optimism.

Developing a chronic disease in addition to an existing mental disorder may reduce independent functioning, limit access to treatment options and worsen psychiatric symptoms.

The incidence of myocardial infarction is increased 4–5 times after an episode of major depression.

Physical symptoms can also be a consequence of emotional dysfunction, including non-epileptic seizures and complex pain syndromes.

Medication can mimic or contribute to symptoms of a mental disorder:

- *Steroids* affect mood.
- *Anticholinergic* medications affect cognition.
- *Beta-blockers* are associated with depression.

Any prescription of psychotropic medication must also consider the potential for adverse effects:

- *SSRIs* may cause hyponatraemia and increased risk of bleeding.
- *Antipsychotics* may cause metabolic syndrome and increased risk of falls.
- *Benzodiazepines* and *hypnotics* may cause respiratory depression.

Secondary and reversible dementias **are listed here:**

V: vitamin deficiency (thiamine, B1, B6, B12, folate and iron).
A: autoimmune (cerebral vasculitis, systemic lupus erythematosus).
N: normal pressure hydrocephalus and neoplasia.
I: infection (Creutzfeldt-Jakob disease, herpes simplex encephalitis, prion diseases, tertiary syphilis, HIV/AIDS).
S: substance abuse and serum abnormalities (hyperammonaemia, uraemia, Wilson's disease).
H: Huntington's disease, hormone disturbances (hypothyroidism, hyperparathyroidism) and haematomas (chronic subdural).
E: electrolyte disturbances (hyponatraemia, hypokalaemia, hypocalcaemia, hypercalcaemia).
D: depression (pseudodementia) and drugs (anticholinergics, steroids, benzodiazepines).

- **Alcohol-related brain damage** presents most commonly in people in their 40–50s.
  Korsakoff amnesia is a form of retrograde and anterograde amnesia, usually a sequela of Wernicke's encephalopathy (triad of *ophthalmoplegia, ataxia* and *acute confusion*) as a result of *thiamine* deficiency, most commonly seen in alcoholics or the severely malnourished.
  The neurotoxic effects of heavy and chronic alcohol consumption can affect the limbic system and frontal lobes, with consequences for executive functioning and emotional reasoning.
  Memory impairment is typically autobiographical resulting in *confabulation*.
  A period of abstinence can partially or fully reverse the cognitive impairment.
- **Vitamin B12 deficiency** is usually due to poor dietary intake or malabsorption from Coeliac's disease or bowel resection. Cognitive impairment is a consequence, amongst many other symptoms, and can improved with B12 replacement.
- **Folate deficiency** and **iron deficiency** can influence cognition in the elderly, independently of anaemia, and replacement is recommended.
- **Normal pressure hydrocephalus** (NPH) is a triad of *gait ataxia, urinary incontinence* and *cognitive impairment* (usually frontal lobe-related with

sparing of memory and orientation) associated with progressive *ventricular dilatation* (seen via brain imaging).

Cerebrospinal fluid pressure is slightly raised or normal.

Dementia is potentially reversible with prompt surgical placement of a ventriculoperitoneal shunt.

- **Neurosyphilis** is an infection of the central nervous system by *Treponema pallidum*. Cognitive impairment is a neuropsychiatric consequence of **tertiary syphilis**, where there has been damage to the brain in the advanced stages of the disease. Its prevalence has reduced with the use of antibiotic treatments for the bacterial cause.

- **HIV-associated dementia** can present with a range of severities, from mild cognitive impairment to severe dementia. Highly active antiretroviral therapy treatment can allow some reversibility.

- **Prion diseases** are caused by insoluble misfolded proteins, which cause *spongiform encephalopathies*, a group of transmissible dementias. All forms are rare, with the most common being **Creutzfeldt-Jakob Disease** (CJD).

CJD is caused by an infectious prion protein, PrP^{Sc}, the accumulation of which leads to rapidly progressive neurodegeneration and focal brain atrophy (worse in frontal lobes and cerebellum).

Presenting features include rapidly progressive dementia, myoclonus, ataxia, dysarthria and postural rigidity, followed by death, usually within 12 months.

Median age at death is 68 years.

The reason for 85% of cases is unknown (sporadic CJD), whereas 7.5% of cases are inherited in an autosomal dominant manner (familial CJD), and 5% are from exposure to infected tissue (acquired CJD).

Definitive diagnosis requires a biopsy of brain tissue. Electroencephalography (EEG), cerebrospinal fluid (CSF) analysis and magnetic resonance imaging (MRI) can all support the diagnosis, as shown in Table 4.4.

Table 4.4 Tests in CJD

Investigation modality	Characteristic finding
EEG	*Generalised periodic sharp wave complexes.*
CSF	*Elevated levels of 14–3–3 protein.*
MRI	*High signal intensity bilaterally in the caudate nucleus and putamen.*
Biopsy	*Spongiform degeneration and gliosis throughout grey matter.*

Variant CJD is a specific form acquired from bovine spongiform encephalopathy transmitted from cattle.

It typically affects *males in their 20s*, with a slightly *longer duration* of illness and absence of EEG findings, instead with '*pulvinar sign*' of *symmetrical high signal intensities* on axial FLAIR MRI being a diagnostic criterion.

Diagnosis can also be performed using a *tonsillar biopsy of lymphoid tissue*.

Huntington's disease is an *autosomal dominant* inherited neurodegenerative disorder caused by the expansion of CAG trinucleotide repeats on the Huntington gene.

Cognitive impairment with mood changes are usually the earliest presenting signs, beginning at age 30–50 and progressing to manifest as coordination difficulties and a choreiform gait with dementia.

Pseudodementia is where the severity of depressive features is the cause for the cognitive impairment and can be treated by treating the depression.

Prevalence/incidence, clinical features, differential diagnosis, aetiology, management and prognosis of the following disorders occurring in late life

Dementia prevalence in individuals aged over 60 is estimated at 5.6–7.6% worldwide, 4.6% in Central Europe and 8.7% in North Africa and the Middle East.

Worldwide, more than 46 million people were estimated to be living with dementia in 2015, and this figure is expected to rise to 131.5 million in 2050.[7]

Worldwide, the annual incidence of new dementia cases is estimated at over 9.9 million. 49% of the total cases occur in Asia, 25% in Europe, 18% in the Americas and 8% in Africa.

The incidence of dementia doubles with every 6.3 years of age from 60 (3.9 per 1000) to 90+ (104.8 per 1000).

In the UK, 7.1% of all people over the age of 65 have dementia. 5.2% of dementia diagnoses are in individuals under 65 years old (42,000 people).

Dementia can be defined as a syndrome due to *disease of the brain*, usually of *chronic or progressive* nature, in which there is *impairment of more than 1 cognitive domain*, including memory, language, fluency, complex attention, executive function, visuospatial, perceptual and social cognition accompanied by *impairment of function*.

Dementia is a clinical syndrome suggesting a range of possible diagnoses; the UK prevalence of each is shown in Table 4.5.

Table 4.5 Prevalence of dementia subtypes[8]

Subtype of dementia	UK prevalence
Alzheimer's disease	62%
Vascular dementia	17%
Mixed dementia	10%
Lewy body dementia	4%
Frontotemporal dementia	2%
Parkinson's dementia	2%
Other	3%

Table 4.6 Clinical features of primary dementias

	Alzheimer's disease	*Vascular dementia*	*Lewy body dementia*	*Frontotemporal dementia*
Disease progression	Gradual/ progressive.	'step-wise'	Progressive with cognitive fluctuations.	Gradual, progressive or variable.
Cognitive domains commonly involved	Episodic memory, language, fluency, executive function, complex attention.	Variable depending on site of lesion. Semantic memory, language, fluency, executive function, complex attention, visuospatial.	Perceptual, visuospatial, attentional, executive (relative sparing of short-term recall).	Social cognition, executive function, attention, language.
Impairment of function	YES	YES	YES	YES

Various objective assessment scales are used in assessment of dementia, as outlined in Table 4.7.

Table 4.7 Objective assessment scales used in dementia

	Maximum total	*Cut-off*	*Findings*
Abbreviated Mental Test Score (AMTS)	10	≤ 8 suggests further assessment necessary.	Memory and orientation.
Mini Mental State Examination (MMSE)	30	≤ 24	Orientation, attention, Memory, language, visuospatial (no measure of frontal lobe function).
Montreal Cognitive Assessment (MoCA)	30	≤ 25	Visuospatial/executive function, language, memory, attention, abstraction, orientation. (includes frontal lobe function).
Dementia Rating Scale (DRS)	54	0–18 – Mild 19–36 – Moderate 37–54 – Severe	Measure the stage of dementia through memory, orientation, judgement/problem solving, community affairs, home/hobbies and personal care.

(Continued)

Table 4.7 (Continued)

	Maximum total	Cut-off	Findings
Addenbrooke's Cognitive Examination (ACE)	100	≤88 (sensitivity = 1.0; specificity = 0.96) ≤82 (sensitivity = 0.93; specificity = 1.0)	Attention, memory, fluency, language, visuospatial.
Cambridge Cognition Examination (Camcog)	Maximum score of 104, from 67 items.	<80 indicates dementia	Comprehensive. 40 minutes to complete. Assesses orientation, language, memory, praxis, attention, abstract thinking, perception and calculation.
Clock drawing test	Subject asked to draw a clock, with numbers, placing hands at 'ten minutes past eleven'.		Demonstrates visuospatial abilities, numerical sequencing and executive function.
Neuropsychiatric Inventory (NPI)	96 12 domains scored by severity (0–3), caregiver distress (0–5)		Assessment of non-cognitive symptoms: delusions, hallucinations, aggression, depression, anxiety, elation, apathy, disinhibition, irritability, motor, appetite.

Mild cognitive impairment (MCI) is a heterogenous clinical syndrome where cognitive abilities are below that expected for age, but without impairment of function.

In some cases, this is a prodrome to neurodegenerative disease, with 5–15% rate of progression to dementia per year.

Other causes include major mental illness (pseudodementia), poor glycaemic control, cerebrovascular disease, medications and functional cognitive disorder.

50% remain stable at 5 years.

Alzheimer's disease (AD)[20]

AD is the biggest single cause of dementia, typically occurring sporadically and after the age of 65, termed 'late-onset'.

Additionally, familial clusters of AD can occur with 3 recognised gene mutations, where presentation is earlier (30–50 years):

- Amyloid precursor protein (APP) – chromosome 21.
- Presenilin 1 (PSEN1) – chromosome 14.
- Presenilin 2 (PSEN2) – chromosome 1.

Sporadic late-onset AD develops as a result of genetic (70%) and environmental factors (30%), as shown in Table 4.8 with *APOE4* (chromosome 19) being the major genetic risk factor in adults irrespective of APOE genotype (11% for men, 14% for women).

Increasing age, Down's syndrome and family history are also established risk factors of AD, with female sex, head injury and declining oestrogen levels post-menopause all probable risk factors.

Possible protective factors include: APOE2, non-steroidal inflammatory drugs (NSAIDs), oestrogen, vitamin E, high premorbid education and physical activity.

The lifetime risk of developing AD where a first-degree relative has been diagnosed is 15–19%, compared to 5% in controls.

Table 4.8 Risk factors for Alzheimer's disease

Genetic	Environmental
APOE3 & 4 heterozygotes (increases lifetime risk by 20–30%)	Early life formal schooling (increases lifetime risk by 8%)
	Mid-life hearing loss (increases lifetime risk by 9%) Mid-life hypertension (increases lifetime risk by 2%)
APOE4 homozygotes (increases lifetime risk by >50%)	Mid-life obesity (increases lifetime risk by 1%)
	Smoking (increases lifetime risk by 5%) Depression (increases lifetime risk by 4%)
Multiple common genetic variants	Physical inactivity (increases lifetime risk by 3%)
conferring small increased risk	Low social contact (increases lifetime risk by 2%) Diabetes (increases lifetime risk by 1%)

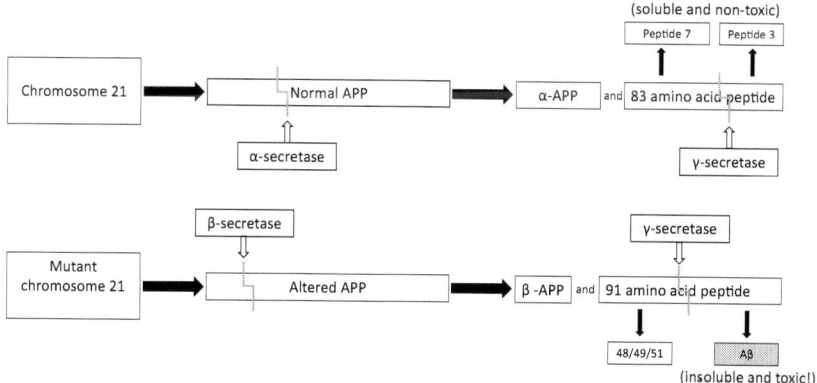

Figure 4.2 The amyloid hypothesis

Amyloid plaques (Aps) and *neurofibrillary tangles* (NFTs) are the main pathological features of AD.

Astrogliosis, microglial activation and *cerebral amyloid angiopathy* (CAA) also have roles in downstream synaptic and neuronal loss, especially *cholinergic neurones* in *nucleus basalis of Meynert* in the basal forebrain, leading to macroscopic atrophy.

Especially in later onset cases, other co-pathologies are also recognised, including vascular disease, Lewy bodies and TAR DNA binding protein-43 (*TDP-43*).

Aps are *extracellular* accumulations of misfolded β-amyloid.

NFTs are *intracellular* aggregates of hyperphosphorylated tau protein.

The *amyloid hypothesis* (Figure 4.2) describes the production of misfolded β-amyloid through the cleavage of amyloid precursor protein (APP) by β- and γ-secretase, where production of pathological β-amyloid is insoluble and toxic. However, it is noted that this hypothesis is complicated by the knowledge that significant β-amyloid deposition can occur without AD symptoms.

Where the direct mechanism linking β-amyloid, tau and AD is unclear, studies suggest that the innate immune system has a role through AD risk genes involved in immune system pathways and neuroinflammation via microglia.

The *amyloid cascade hypothesis* proposes that abnormal processing of amyloid leads to abnormal processing of tau proteins to form NFTs. Hence, the extent of NFT progression is a better correlate of clinical severity than the presence of amyloid plaques.

Braak staging outlines the classical progression of NFTs in Alzheimer's disease:

Stage I–II   = mild or severe alteration of the *transentorhinal* layer.
Stage III–IV   = involvement of *limbic* regions including hippocampus.
Stages V–VI   = involvement of the cortex and temporal lobes.

Typically, AD presents in elderly patients as a gradual and progressive loss of episodic memory alongside other cognitive domains. The course of decline should be at least 6 months with clear consciousness and without evidence of other brain disease which might be affecting cognition.

Atypical subtypes of AD are outlined in Table 4.9.

A diagnosis of *probable AD* can be made for a typical clinical syndrome without clear pathological evidence (brain imaging or biomarkers).

A diagnosis of *possible AD* can be made for an atypical clinical syndrome without clear pathological evidence, but with no alternative diagnosis.

Evidence of AD pathology can help to establish the diagnosis with confidence.

Table 4.9 Atypical Alzheimer's disease subtypes

Posterior cortical atrophy (PCA)	Tau pathology is focused on parietal and occipital lobes. Visuospatial and perceptual problems are prominent with dyspraxia. Memory is relatively preserved.
Logopenic progressive aphasia (LPA)	LPA is a variant of primary progressive aphasia due to AD (usually language variant dementias are classified under frontotemporal dementias). Presentation is with anomia, prominent word finding difficulty, pauses and executive dysfunction.
Frontal variant AD (fvAD)	Presents similarly to behavioural variants of frontotemporal dementia with prominent personality and behavioural changes, most notably apathy, disinhibition, loss of self-awareness and loss of empathy.

Computed tomography (CT):

* Rule out other causes – NPH, neoplastic lesions, trauma.
* Demonstrate characteristic cortical atrophy.

MRI

* Assessment of focal volume loss in characteristic locations in progressed AD.
* Mesial temporal lobe atrophy.
* Temporoparietal cortical atrophy.
* *Medial temporal atrophy* (MTA) score is used to distinguish MCI from AD. Under 75 years with score ≥ 2 is abnormal; 75+ years a score ≥ 3 is abnormal.
* *Entorhinal cortical atrophy* (ERICA) score is used to distinguish healthy controls from patients with AD. Scores range from 0–3 with scores ≥ 2 highly specific for AD.

F-18 fluorodeoxyglucose (FDG) PET:

* Glucose hypometabolism in characteristic locations, with sparing elsewhere.
* Temporoparietal, praecuneus and posterior cingulate regions.
* Usually symmetrical, may be asymmetrical in early stages.

Amyloid PET:

* Demonstrates tracer binding to β-amyloid.
* Useful in excluding AD, as amyloid deposition occurs in healthy patients.

Cerebrospinal fluid *biomarkers*:

• It is possible to measure CSF levels of β-amyloid (Aβ42), total tau and phosphorylated tau.

Non-cognitive symptoms, also termed behavioural and psychological symptoms of dementia (BPSD) or neuropsychiatric symptoms are common. These are categorised in the NPI.

BPSDs often lead to a high burden for carers, particularly irritability, agitation, sleep disturbances, anxiety, apathy and delusion.

2 classes of medication are licensed as treatments for AD:

Acetylcholinesterase inhibitors (AchEis) – donepezil, rivastigmine and galantamine are licensed for *mild to moderate AD* where they have a modest benefit in slowing the progression of cognitive decline. They have no effect on neurodegeneration. By inhibiting the breakdown of acetylcholine, they work to potentiate its level and duration of action as a neurotransmitter. Main side effects: bradycardia (pulse checks are necessary), headaches, syncope, gastrointestinal: nausea, diarrhoea, anorexia. Donepezil is dosed once daily. Rivastigmine can be administered as a transdermal patch.

NMDA antagonists – *memantine* is licensed for moderate to severe AD, or mild AD where AchEis have not been tolerated. These may have an effect on neurodegeneration by reducing excessive glutamate production, thought to be neurotoxic in AD. Requires dose adjustment in cases of renal failure. Main side effects: drowsiness, dizziness, headaches, constipation. Caution should be taken in patients with epilepsy.

Risperidone is the only medication licensed for treatment of non-cognitive symptoms of dementia.

It should only be used where non-pharmacological approaches are unsuccessful and there is a risk of significant harm or distress.

Patients and carers should be made aware that risperidone in dementia has an increased risk of stroke and premature death.

The average life expectancy from diagnosis of AD is 8–10 years. 40% of these years are spent in the severe stage.

At age 80, 75% of people with AD will live in a nursing home, compared to 4% of healthy controls.

In 2019, AD was listed as the sixth-leading cause of death in the United States.

Vascular dementia (VaD)[21]:

VaD, the second most common type of dementia, is diagnosed where cognitive impairment is caused by cerebral ischaemia from thrombosis, embolism or haemorrhage.

It may be due to a single large infarction, multiple transient ischaemic attacks (TIAs) in *multi-infarct dementia* or *subcortical vascular dementia* where there are vascular risk factors and foci of ischaemic destruction in the deep white matter.

The clinical course is variable, with acute onset following a single infarction, more gradual in purely subcortical disease, or step-wise following TIAs.

Diagnosis should demonstrate evidence of cerebrovascular disease with a chronological relationship to the cognitive decline.

Relevant neuroimaging includes CT and MRI, both providing evidence for ischaemic changes, with MRI being more sensitive, specifically for white matter small vessel disease and CAA.

Hachinski index score

Feature	Score
Abrupt onset of symptoms	2
Stepwise deterioration (eg, decline-stability-decline)	1
Fluctuating course	2
Nocturnal confusion	1
Personality relatively preserved	1
Depression	1
Somatic complaints (eg, body aches, chest pain)	1
Emotional lability	1
History or presence of hypertension	1
History of stroke	2
Evidence of coexisting atherosclerosis	1
Focal neurologic symptoms	2
Focal neurologic signs	2

Total score < 4 suggests primary dementia, 4–7 is indeterminate, > 7 suggests VaD

The neurocognitive profile is similar to that of AD but is more variable depending on the location of vascular lesions. Insight is often retained. The classical description applies more closely with subcortical VaD: impaired attention and planning, difficulty with complex activities and disorganised thought, behaviour or emotion.

Risk factors include cardiovascular disease, CAA, sleep apnoea, smoking, physical inactivity, hypercholesterolemia, alcohol excess, family history, APOE4.

Cerebral autosomal dominant arteriopathy with subcortical infarcts and leukoencephalopathy (CADASIL) is an inherited (chromosome 19) form of VaD presenting with recurrent strokes in individuals aged 40–50 with subsequent subcortical dementia and pseudobulbar palsy.

Due to the heterogeneity of causes, there is no single medical treatment for VaD, with approaches instead focussing on optimising of vascular risk factors.

Dementia with Lewy bodies (DLB)[22] is recognised by a triad of fluctuating cognitive impairment and attention, visual hallucinations and parkinsonian features.

Fluctuating cognition is usually a pronounced variation in attention and alertness.

Visual hallucinations (typically of small children or animals) are often well-formed and detailed.

DLB patients are highly sensitive to parkinsonian side effects of antipsychotic medications, with quetiapine and clozapine being the better tolerated.

Short-term recall is relatively preserved, with attention and visuospatial loss more prominent.

The pathological hallmark of Lewy bodies are also seen in Parkinson's disease (PD): *eosinophilic intracytoplasmic neuronal inclusions* made up of *ubiquitin and α-synuclein aggregates.*

The location of degeneration (limbic, brainstem and neocortex) clinically differentiates the presentation from PD.

Diagnostic criteria for probable and possible DLB

Essential feature: progressive cognitive decline of sufficient magnitude to interfere with function

Core clinical features:
Fluctuating cognition - pronounced variations in attention and alertness.
Recurrent visual hallucinations.
REM sleep behaviour disorder
Features of parkinsonism: bradykinesia, rest tremor or rigidity.

Supportive clinical features:
Severe sensitivity to antipsychotic medications; postural instability; repeated falls; syncope or episodic unresponsiveness; severe autonomic dysfunction; hyposmia; hallucinations in other
modalities; systematised delusions; apathy, anxiety and depression.

Indicative biomarkers:
Reduced dopamine transporter uptake in basal ganglia demonstrated by DAT Scan.
Abnormal myocardial scintigraphy.
Polysomnographic confirmation of REM sleep without atonia.

Probable DLB =
a. Two or more core clinical features, with or without the presence of biomarkers, or
b. One core clinical feature, and one or more biomarkers.

Possible DLB =
a. One core clinical feature, with no biomarker evidence, or
b. One indicative biomarkers but there are no core clinical features.

Rivastigmine is licensed for treatment of DLB and shows efficacy in delaying the progression of cognitive decline, as well as benefits in treating hallucinations and delusions.

Lifetime survival from the point of diagnosis is 8 years on average.

Parkinson's disease dementia

In PD, the site of Lewy body degeneration is focused on subcortical structures (substantia nigra, caudate, putamen and globus pallidus), which explains the clinical neurological features. Bradyphrenia is a common non-motor feature of PD and 10% of affected individuals progress to dementia. Where this progression occurs >12 months after the motor symptoms, it is termed PD dementia, rather than DLB.

Treatment of PD with dopamine agonists is associated with delusions and hallucinations.

Frontotemporal dementia (FTD)

FTD includes 3 subtypes: behavioural variant FTD (bvFTD) classically known as Pick's disease, language variant FTD or primary progressive aphasia (PPA) and corticobasal syndrome (CBS), as shown in Figure 4.3. Presentation typically occurs earlier than in other dementias, before 60 years of age.

Clinical presentation is typically focused on behavioural changes such as apathy, emotional lability or repetitiveness, as well as personality changes such as impulsivity, disinhibition and social inappropriateness. Memory problems are less prominent than in AD.

CT or MRI scans will demonstrate bilateral asymmetrical atrophy of the frontal and temporal lobes, with 'knife blade atrophy' often used to describe the sharpened appearance of the gyri.

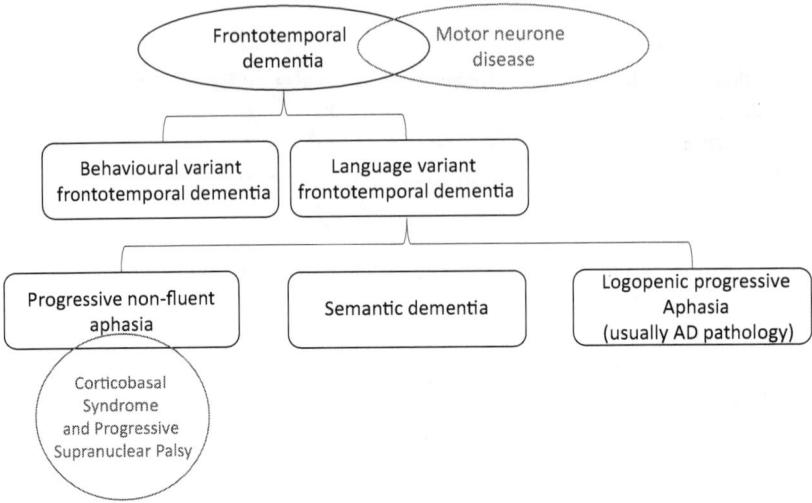

Figure 4.3 Subtypes of frontotemporal dementia

FTD has clinical overlap with motor neurone disease though shared pathology related to ubiquitin and transactive response DNA binding protein of 43 kDa (TDP 43).

In *bvFTD*, the most common form of FTD, the neurodegeneration is prominent in the early stages of the disease in the frontal lobes, with a corresponding presentation profile where personality and behavioural changes precede memory deficits.

In PPA, a decline in language function is most prominent initially, with other cognitive domains preserved until later in the disease when behavioural changes develop, as in bvFTD.

In a 'semantic' variant of PPA, speech is fluent but with loss of meaning of words and declining vocabulary.

In progressive non-fluent aphasia, speech is hesitant with frequent grammatical mistakes and speech errors. Comprehension of words in preserved. *Left hemispheric frontal atrophy* is seen on imaging, preferably using positron emission tomography (PET).

Corticobasal syndrome usually features asymmetrical parkinsonism with severe limb apraxia, falls and myoclonus. Most patients will also develop dementia with progressive non-fluent aphasia.

Kluver-Bucy syndrome is seen in progressed FTD where bilateral damage to the anterior temporal lobes is associated with a tendency to put inedible objects in the mouth and engage in inappropriate sexual behaviour.

Progressive supranuclear palsy is a syndrome of supranuclear ophthalmoplegia, pseudobulbar palsy and axial dystonia, which is often not recognised until a year after initial presentation.

Earlier signs include loss of balance with falls, bradykinesia, dysarthria, cognitive impairment, personality changes and vertical gaze palsy. It may be mistaken for DLB.

Delirium[23] is an acute change in attention, awareness and cognition due to an underlying medical condition, and is not better explained by an established neurocognitive disorder. It occurs with 'clouded consciousness' and disorientation. The onset of symptoms is rapid (usually less than a week of the precipitating cause) and resolving quickly, but potentially taking months.

Dementia and frailty are known to be increased risk and possible causes are varied (Figure 4.3) with no cause is determined in 5–20% of cases.

Hyperactive delirium presents with increased motor activity, agitation, hallucinations and behavioural changes.

Hypoactive delirium presents with reduced motor activity and lethargy, being less readily recognised with a poorer prognosis.

Pathophysiology is understood to involve acute neuronal dysfunction and network disintegration, specifically affecting the ascending arousal systems via cholinergic drive from the tegmentum to the thalamus.

A characteristic EEG pattern of *generalised slowing* is demonstrated.

Prevalence amongst hospital inpatients can be up to 23%.

Causes of delirium (PINCHSME):

Pain.
Infection (UTI, pneumonia, encephalitis, etc.).
Nutrition – hunger, thiamine/B12 deficiency.
Constipation.
Hydration.
Stroke and surgery.
Medication (alcohol/withdrawal, sedatives, anticholinergics, etc.).
Endocrine (thyroid, adrenal, glycaemia), electrolyte imbalance (sodium, calcium) and environment change.

Rating scales in delirium include:

Single question in delirium (SqiD) – 'Is this patient more confused than before?'
Delirium rating scale (DRS) – allows for distinguishing between delirium and dementia.
Confusion assessment method (CAM) – highly sensitive and specific, permits a diagnosis.
Mini Mental State Examination (MMSE) – is not specific to delirium but can demonstrate changes over time with consecutive assessments.

Table 4.10 Comparing delirium and dementia

	Delirium	Dementia
Onset	Sudden, with a definite beginning.	Slow and gradual, with uncertain beginning point.
Duration	Days to weeks, possibly months.	Usually permanent.
Cause	Almost always another condition.	Usually a chronic brain disorder.
Course	Usually reversible.	Slowly progressive.
Attention	Greatly impaired.	Unimpaired until dementia has become severe.
Level of consciousness	Variably impaired.	Unimpaired until dementia has become severe.
Use of language	Slow, often incoherent and inappropriate.	Occasional difficulty finding the right word.
Need for medical attention	Immediate.	Required but less urgent.

Primary management of delirium is through treatment of the underlying cause, optimising the environment of the individual, addressing any sensory deficits (hearing/eyesight) and ensuring hydration, nutrition, normal bowel movements and pain management.

Use of medication is rarely appropriate and should only be used where there is a significant risk of distress that is not amenable with non-pharmacological approaches.

Haloperidol is NICE-approved, but evidence suggests antipsychotics worsen outcomes in delirium and lower hospital survival in older patients.

Benzodiazepines can paradoxically increase agitation through disinhibition and may increase risk of falls in the elderly. They do have a role if the cause of delirium is due to substance withdrawal.

Depression[24] in the elderly is complicated by comorbid physical conditions, cognitive decline and higher incidence of significant life events or losses.

Depression in the elderly may be recurrence of an early-onset (before 65 years of age) depression or a late-onset disorder, without previous history before 65 years of age. These subtypes are not recognised in ICD or DSM.

Diagnosis is also complicated by a high degree of alexithymia and somatisation which may mask the mental disorder.

Patient reports of 'not coping', anxiety or irritability are more common than depressed mood, and are seen in 80% of late-onset depression cases, rendering subjective reports of depressed mood as not essential for diagnosis.

Physical features may be more readily expressed: poor sleep, reduced appetite, loss of energy. Somatisation is often observed in late-onset depression, but comorbid physical diagnoses are also commonly identified (46%) in screening of psychiatric referrals.

Cognitive deficits are also common in the depressed elderly, sometimes to the extent of pseudodementia, and will require full cognitive assessment to rule out true dementia.

Suicidal ideas are common, as are suicidal acts, with risk factors including being unmarried, poor subjective health, disability, pain, sensory impairment and living in a nursing home.

Behavioural changes are also not uncommon: food refusal, non-medical incontinence, theatrical 'falls'.

These differences from depression in working-age people are reflected in the geriatric depression scale (GDS) shown in the following box.

Geriatric Depression Scale

Are you basically satisfied with your life?	Yes/No
Have you dropped many of your activities and interests?	Yes/No
Do you feel that your life is empty?	Yes/No
Do you often get bored?	Yes/No
Are you in good spirits most of the time?	Yes/No
Are you afraid that something bad is going to happen to you?	Yes/No
Do you feel happy most of the time?	Yes/No
Do you often feel helpless?	Yes/No
Do you prefer to stay at home, rather than go out and do new things?	Yes/No
Do you feel you have more problems with memory than most?	Yes/No
Do you think it is wonderful to be alive?	Yes/No
Do you feel pretty worthless the way you are now?	Yes/No
Do you feel full of energy?	Yes/No
Do you feel that your situation is hopeless?	Yes/No
Do you think that most people are better off than you are?	Yes/No

(Number of Yes responses:
0-4 normal, 5-9 Mild depression, 10-15 More severe depression)

The prevalence of depression in the elderly is similar to that in people of working age (1–3%). The proportion of older people who would be considered as needing treatment is 10–15%, increasing to 30–40% in residential settings.

A diagnosis of cancer, cardiovascular disease or central nervous system disorders (stroke, PD, dementia) are all recognised as strong risk factors for the subsequent development of depression.

Risk factors for late-onset depression:

- Physical illness.
- Social isolation and loneliness.

- Recent bereavement.
- Hearing difficulties.
- Female gender (7:3 F:M).

Late-onset depression is associated with:

- Increased incidence of structural cerebral abnormalities.
- Decreased likelihood of a family history of depression.
- Poor treatment response, as shown by longer hospital stays and more residual symptoms.
- Increased risk of progression to dementia.
- Earlier mortality.

Treatment of depression in the elderly:

NICE guidelines do not differentiate management of depression for older and younger adults.

First-line treatment for mild to moderate depression includes offering patients the choice of:

- Guided self-help.
- Group or individual talking therapies (cognitive behavioural therapy [CBT], interpersonal therapy or psychodynamic therapy).
- Selective serotonin reuptake inhibitors (SSRIs).

For moderate to severe depression, a combination of antidepressant mediations and CBT is recommended.

Antidepressants have higher efficacy than placebos in the elderly, with a number needed to treat between 4–8[25], similar to other age groups.

In older adults, continuation of antidepressant therapy is associated with a reduced rate of relapse.

Prescribing antidepressants should be specific to older adults:

- Lower starting doses are advised due to differences in pharmacodynamics and tolerability.
- Time to response may take 6–8 weeks.
- SSRIs should be used a first-line therapy due to their relative efficacy and safety profile.
- SSRIs modestly increase the risk of upper gastrointestinal bleeding, particularly when co-administered with aspirin/NSAIDs.
- SSRIs are associated with hyponatraemia.
- Citalopram and escitalopram are associated with a dose-dependant prolongation of the QT-interval, and ECG monitoring is necessary.
- SSRIs, mirtazapine and bupropion do not generally increase the risk of cardiovascular events following myocardial infarction (MI). Tricyclic antidepressants may be associated with an increased risk of MI.

Electroconvulsion therapy (ECT) is highly efficacious in severe depression and is well tolerated. It is most commonly used in medication-resistant depression and in urgent and emergency cases such as depressive stupor, high risk of suicide, extreme levels of distress and poor fluid intake.

Bilateral electrode placement ECT is preferable for efficacy and speed of response.

ECT is associated with confusion and cognitive impairment in the elderly, where unilateral electrode placement may be necessary.

Bipolar affective disorder[26] prevalence in older adults has little published evidence. That which exists indicate that community prevalence declines in later life: 1-year prevalence of 0.1% in individuals over 65 years old (compared to 1.4% in young adults and 0.4% in middle-aged adults). Inpatient prevalence is estimated at 8–10%.

Little published evidence specifies the prevalence and aetiology in older adults. Treatment is also based on studies carried out in working-age populations.

Studies between early-onset and late-onset bipolar disorder report less familiar risk in late-onset groups, although the age cut-off for 'late-onset' varies from 30–65 years.

In late-onset groups, there is a higher incidence of neurological illness, including cerebrovascular burden and organic brain diseases.

The following conditions are recognised as having a relationship with late-onset mania:

- Cerebrovascular insult.
- Head injury.
- Tumour.
- Medications – antiparkinsonian and steroids.
- CNS infections – HIV and vasculitis.

Few differences have been identified between symptoms in older and younger adults. Presence of psychotic features is similar, with a suggestion that paranoia is more common in older adults.

Studies have inconsistently reported a lower incidence of mixed affective episodes in older adults.

First-episode mania in later life is not common and is usually secondary to an organic brain disorder.

Treatment response in late-onset bipolar disorder is not thought to be different from that in early onset, although the incidence of adverse effects is thought to be higher due to differences in pharmacodynamics and medical comorbidity. Treatment with lithium is considered the first line, but with a lower target range of between 0.4–0.6 mmol/L.

Late-life psychosis[27] has a wide range of causes in older adults, making it difficult to distinguish diagnoses. Causes of acute onset include delirium and substance misuse.

Insidious and chronic-onset psychosis may be due to a recurrence of schizophrenia, late-onset schizophrenia (LOS) (onset >40 years of age) or very-late-onset schizophrenia (VLOS) (onset >60 years of age). 3% of schizophrenia diagnoses include onset after age 60. Delusional disorder and psychotic depression also occur in older adults.

Neurodegenerative disorders are also recognised causes of psychotic symptoms.

The term 'paraphrenia' was introduced by Emil Kraepelin in 1913 to describe psychosis in older adults, without an understanding of whether the cause was primary mental illness or secondary to organic or neurodegenerative disorders.

The lifetime prevalence of schizophrenia in older adults is 0.3%, compared to 1.0% in people aged 45–65. Women present more commonly than men.

10% of older people with an early-onset schizophrenia (EOS) diagnosis achieve sustained remission of psychotic symptoms. Otherwise, the illness course is mostly unchanged apart from some improvement in positive symptoms, higher prevalence of negative symptoms and higher prevalence of cognitive deficits (learning, abstraction and cognitive flexibility), which remain stable.

Risk factors and clinical presentation for LOS are similar to those of EOS. Rate of cognitive decline in LOS is not different to that in EOS, hence it is considered a neurodevelopment disorder similar to EOS, rather than a neurodegenerative disorder.

Patients with VLOS have higher rates of marriage, higher premorbid education, a favourable response to risperidone and more pronounced cerebellar atrophy, suggesting it is a neurodegenerative process.

Clinically, VLOS presents with less thought disorder and fewer negative symptoms.

Partition delusions are commonly described in late-onset psychosis, with the individual believing they are being harmed by spying, stealing or noxious substance across a partition such as a wall or ceiling.

Deteriorating hearing or eyesight, and social isolation are recognised as risk factors for late-onset psychosis.

Of the limited available evidence, treatment of LOS and VLOS is similar to that of EOS, with atypical antipsychotics being preferred due to their side-effect profile. Age-related dose adjustments are necessary, taking into account differences in pharmacodynamics and comorbidity.

The risk of developing tardive dyskinesia is significantly increased.

Antipsychotics are associated with a significant increase in risk of stroke and mortality in patients with dementia, which must be considered where cognitive impairment is being considered.

Extrapyramidal side effects with the introduction of antipsychotics, particularly at low doses, may be the first evidence for DLB.

Anxiety disorders[28]

The prevalence of anxiety disorders in older adults is estimated as between 3.2% to 14.2%, depending on the age criteria, time frame and definition of 'anxiety disorders' used. This is generally lower than the prevalence in working-age adults, but is still relatively high.

Table 4.11 Prevalence of specific anxiety disorders

Specific phobia	3.1–10.2%
Generalised anxiety disorder	1.2–7.8%
Social phobia	0.6–2.3%
Obsessive-compulsive disorder	0.8–1.5%
Panic disorder	0.1–1.0%
Post-traumatic stress disorder	0.4–1.0%

Fewer than 1% of individuals will develop an anxiety disorder in later life. Risk factors for experiencing an anxiety disorder as an older adult include:

* Being female.
* Medical comorbidity.
* Being single, divorced or separated.
* Low educational status.
* Impaired subjective health.
* Stressful life events.
* Physical limitation in activities of daily living.
* Adverse childhood events.
* Neuroticism.

Older adults report experiencing less burden of negative emotional states: depression, anxiety/guilt, hostility or shyness.

The focus for anxiety is often regarding health, disability and burden on others. Anxiety is less often related to work, finances and family.

Anxiety confers an increased risk of mortality after cardiac surgery and is also a risk factor for developing coronary heart disease.

The incidence of anxiety, particularly panic disorder with agoraphobia, is higher amongst chronic obstructive pulmonary disease (COPD) patients.

Postural disturbance, dizziness and falls all increase the incidence of anxiety, and often lead to a restriction of daily activities.

The relationship between anxiety disorders and cognitive decline is complex. Anxiety can be a cause or contributing factor for MCI and may be a predictor for subsequent cognitive impairment.

Of patients with MCI and anxiety, an estimated 83% go on to develop dementia after 3 years.

The prevalence of anxiety disorders in patients with dementia is 3.3%, similar to that in older people without dementia.

Antidepressants are effective treatments for anxiety in older adults, with similar response rates to those in working-age people and similar tolerability.

CBT is also effective for treating older adults with anxiety but may require some age-appropriate adjustments in the approach.

Substance misuse[29]

Substance misuse in the elderly may occur without the person experiencing cravings or insight into the potential harms.

Psychomotor performance, cognition and deteriorating coordination with increase in falls may be noted.

Intoxication or withdrawal may be associated with changes in alertness, sudden changes in mood or aggression.

Self-neglect and malnutrition may be consequences of substance misuse in the elderly.

Blood test abnormalities may be noted, as in Table 4.12.

Table 4.12 Blood test abnormalities in substance misuse

Blood test abnormality	Associated substance misuse
Liver function tests	General substance misuse
Hypercholesterolaemia	General substance misuse
Hyperuricaemia	General substance misuse
Hypoglycaemia	General substance misuse
Low platelets	Alcohol misuse
Microcytic anaemia	Alcohol misuse
Low folate	Alcohol misuse
Γ-glutamyltransferase	Alcohol misuse

The amount of alcohol that is likely to cause harm in older adults in less than that in people of working age due to pharmacokinetics, comorbid physical illness and medication interactions.

70% of alcohol misuse in the elderly occurs in those with a history of alcohol misuse as a younger adult. A positive family history is also more common.

Late-onset 'reactors' develop alcohol misuse after 50 years of age in response to a life stressor and are often in a higher income bracket.

Treatment of alcohol misuse is broadly similar to that in working-age people:

• Chlordiazepoxide is usually the preferred treatment for alcohol withdrawal.
• Disulfiram and acamprosate have a role in maintaining abstinence. It should be noted that disulfiram can cause delirium and is contraindicated in various medical conditions.
• Thiamine should be prescribed to prevent Wernicke-Korsakoff's syndrome.

Lifetime prevalence of substance misuse in older adults is 1.6%, lower than that for working-age people. Dependant use of recreational drugs in >60-year-olds has a prevalence of <1%.

Short Michigan alcoholism screening test
(geriatric version)

1. Do you ever underestimate how much you drink?
2. After drinking do you ever skip meals?
3. Does drinking decrease shakes or tremors?
4. Does alcohol make you not remember parts of the day and night?
5. Do you drink to relax or calm your nerves?
6. Do you drink to take your mind off problems?
7. Have you ever increased your drinking after a loss in your life?
8. Has a doctor or nurse said they're worried about your drinking?
9. Have you ever made rules to manage your drinking?
10. When lonely does drinking help?

Answering 'yes' to two or more questions suggests further assessment for alcohol misuse is necessary.

Suicide and attempted suicide in old age[30]

In general, completed suicide rates across the world rise to a peak in old age. Interestingly, in the United States and Canada, the peak is in mid-life and reduces thereafter, with the exception of white males in United States, who exhibit a second rise from 70–74 years, and of black males, where there are 2 peaks: in early adulthood and again in old age.

Incidents of deliberate self-harm and attempted suicide decrease in frequency with advancing age, and should therefore be treated with greater significance.

Attempted suicide in females is more common than males (ratio 3:2) but accounting for generations in older age, the incidence is proportionally 1:1, with males more likely to successfully end their life.

Most attempted suicides are by deliberate drug overdose (benzodiazepines, analgesics and antidepressants), followed by hanging and suffocation.

Ideas of life being hopeless and wishing to die can occur without low mood, but mental illness is the biggest risk factor for suicide in older adults, present in approximately 90% of cases.

Risk factors for suicide in older adults:

- Mental illness.
- Being unmarried or recently separated.
- Substance misuse.

- Comorbid physical illness and disability.
- Pain.
- Sensory impairment.
- Social isolation.
- Living in a nursing or care home.
- Recent bereavement of grief reaction.

Psychiatric aspects of personality in old age[31]

It is recognised that personality traits can evolve with age; specifically, cautiousness, obsessiveness and compulsivity can increase with age.

Depressive illness is likely to present with dependant and avoidant personality traits.

Psychotic depression is likely to present with hypochondriacal personality traits.

Dementia is commonly associated with coarsening of pre-existing personality traits in addition to behavioural changes that are recognised in BPSD and FTD.

The prevalence of personality disorders in older adults is estimated at 10–17% in the general population and at 58% in care and nursing home residents.

A diagnosis is more likely in individuals who are male, younger and more highly educated.

Prevalence rates for personality disorder in a study considering all 10 possible diagnosis were highest for obsessive-compulsive personality disorder (7.6%). Borderline personality disorder prevalence was 3.2%. Dependent personality disorder prevalence was the lowest, at 0.26%.

Diagnosis of personality disorder should ideally be carried out using an objective screening method using multiple sources of information.

Recognition of the disorder is necessary due to high levels of suffering, poorer functioning, treatment rejection and non-adherence.

Higher rates of generalised anxiety and substance misuse are recognised in the presence of personality disorder.

Diogenes syndrome

Known as 'senile squalor syndrome' presents with severe self-neglect in older adults, usually living in squalor due to hoarding behaviour, without understanding of the concern from others, and resistant to help that is offered.

It often occurs in individuals who have had an eccentric or reclusive personality through their life.

Psychotherapy with older adults

It is important to cautiously avoid therapeutic pessimism with older adults. Psychotherapy is as effective, if not more so, as in younger adults.

Thematic changes in therapy specific to older adults include primarily that of death and loss: relationships, employment, status, independence, physical ability and health.

Changes in cognition must also be considered when adapting therapeutic approaches.

Invariably, the therapist will be younger than the patient and the potential for transference reaction and envy must be recognised.

CBT has the strongest evidence base for treatment of depression in older adults, and as such is most commonly used.

Interpersonal therapy has good evidence for relapse prevention in depression.

Family therapy is popular and effective for depression and dementia.

Bereavement and adjustment disorders[32]

Likelihood of bereavement, a grief reaction to the loss of a loved one, is more likely as people age.

Bereavement is associated with weight loss, increased rate of illness and loss of function. These outcomes resolve with the grief reaction, usually after 2–3 months.

John Bowlby described the stages of grief, observing that people can go back and forth between the stages and that there is no specific time frame to move from one to another:

- Phase 1 – Shock and disbelief: first few days
- Phase 2 – Preoccupation, yearning and anger: first few weeks
- Phase 3 – Disorganisation, despair and acceptance of loss: several months
- Phase 4 – Resolution: 1–2 years

The Kubler-Ross model of grief stages can be remembered as **DABDA**:

Denial > **A**nger > **B**argaining > **D**epression > **A**cceptance

Complicated (abnormal) grief:

> A delayed grief reaction occurs where there is a marked lack of grief in the first 2 weeks following the loss, as the individual consciously or unconsciously makes an effort to avoid painful emotions.

A prolonged grief reaction is where grief related symptoms, including the following, persist long after the death (>6 months). Treatment should be considered at this stage, or earlier if suicidal ideas are present.

- Generalised guilt – not just specifically related to the deceased.
- Suicidal thoughts.
- Hallucinations – not of the deceased.
- Feelings of worthlessness.

Table 4.13 Comparison of major depressive disorder and complicated grief[33]

Major depressive disorder	Complicated grief
Pervasive sad mood	Sadness related to missing the deceased
Loss of interest or pleasure in most activities	Strong interest in the deceased maintained
Pervasive sense of guilt	Guilt related to the death or deceased
Low self-esteem	Self-criticism only related to the loss
Suicidal thoughts related to a range of negative emotions and cognitions	Suicidal thoughts focused on not wanting to live without the deceased or a wish to join the deceased
Not seen in depression	Avoidance of situations and people related to reminders of the loss
Not seen in depression	Intense yearning for the person who died

Persistent complex bereavement disorder is now recognised in the DSM-5.

An adjustment disorder is defined as a state of distress and emotional disturbance, severe enough to interfere with functioning, that occurs in response to a significant life event or stressor.

Common stressors that may trigger an adjustment disorder in the elderly include:

- Bereavement.
- Retirement.
- Migration or a significant move.
- Medical illness or disability.
- Loss of mobility or independence.

Sleep disorder in later life

As people age, sleep architecture naturally changes:

- Total sleep time is reduced.
- Sleep efficiency is reduced.
- REM sleep is reduced.

- Slow-wave sleep is reduced.
- Time to sleep onset (latency) is increased.
- REM sleep latency is reduced.
- Time awake during time in bed is increased.

Circadian rhythms may be negatively affected by variable daily schedules, difficulty exercising, and less exposure to natural light.
Medical conditions can affect sleep:

- Pain.
- Cardiac and respiratory conditions – congestive cardiac failure, COPD, obstructive sleep apnoea.
- Real failure and anaemia may affect restless leg syndrome.
- Medications: benzodiazepines, tricyclic antidepressants and beta-blockers all reduce REM sleep; AchEi increase REM sleep.
- Prostatic hypertrophy.
- Dementia, depression and anxiety.

In treating insomnia where no underlying cause has been found, sleep hygiene advice should be the first line. CBT for sleep also has a good evidence base.
Pharmacological options for insomnia include:

- Melatonin agonists.
- Z-drugs where risk of dependence is low – shorter acting zolpidem is preferred (no longer than 2 weeks).
- Benzodiazepines where risk of dependence is low – shorter acting temazepam is preferred (no longer than 2 weeks).
- Sedating antidepressants (mirtazapine) are useful in comorbid depression.

REM behavioural sleep disorder, a type of 'parasomnia', is characterised by dream enactment due to loss of normal muscle atonia during the REM phase of sleep. Activity can be severe with risk of harm to the patient and bed partner.
Prevalence is high in LBD, PD and MSA. It may predate the diagnosis my several years.
Treatment with clonazepam and melatonin are both beneficial.

Psychosexual disorders in old age, including sexuality in physically ill/disabled people, sexuality in institutionalised elderly

A range of physical factors can influence sexual function in older adults:

- Sexual problems are more common: erectile dysfunction, anorgasmia, dyspareunia.

- Medications affecting sexual function are more common: antidepressants, beta-blockers, benzodiazepines, parkinsonian medications.
- Physical conditions which may affect sexual dysfunction are more common: diabetes, cardiovascular disease, cerebrovascular disease, Peyronie's disease, mastectomy, colostomy, prostatectomy or hysterectomy, incontinence.
- Reduced oestrogen levels in women cause vaginal dryness and changes to vaginal anatomy which may make penetration less pleasant.
- Decline in testosterone may decrease sexual desire and response to sexual stimulation.

Inappropriate sexual behaviour may occur in patients with dementia through disinhibition or intimacy seeking. Capacity to consent to sexual activity may also be affected.

References

1. Royal College of Psychiatrists (2018) *Suffering in silence: Age inequality in older people's mental health care*. London: Royal College of Psychiatrists.
2. Nash, A. (2017) *National population projections: 2016-based statistical bulletin*. London: Office for National Statistics (ONS).
3. Age UK (2016) Hidden in plain sight: The unmet mental health needs of older people. *Age UK*. www.ageuk.org.uk/brandpartnerglobal/wiganboroughvpp/hidden_in_plain_sight_older_peoples_mental_health.pdf
4. Bryant C, Jackson H, Ames D (2008) The prevalence of anxiety in older adults: Methodological issues and a review of the literature. *Journal of Affective Disorders*, 109(3), 233–250.
5. Wittenberg R, Hu B, Barraza-Araiza L, Rehill A. (2019) *Projections of older people with dementia and costs of dementia care in the United Kingdom, 2019–2040*. London: London School of Economics.
6. Prince MJ, Wimo A, Guerchet MM, et al. (2015). *World Alzheimer report 2015 – The global impact of Dementia: An analysis of prevalence, incidence, cost and trends*. London: Alzheimer's Disease International, p. 84.
7. Mukadam N, Sommerlad A, Huntley J, Livingston G (2019). Population attributable fractions for risk factors for dementia in low-income and middle-income countries: An analysis using cross-sectional survey data. *The Lancet Global Health*, 7(5), e596–e603.
8. National Collaborating Centre for Mental Health (2021) *The community mental health framework for adults and older adults: Support, care and treatment. Part 1*. London: National Collaborating Centre for Mental Health
9. Criteria for old age psychiatry services in the UK, RCPsych Faculty of the Psychiatry of Old Age; October 2015
10. World Health Organization (2007). *Everybody's business – strengthening health systems to improve health outcomes: WHO's Framework for Action*. Geneva: WHO.
11. Bartels SJ, Dums AR, Oxman TE et al. (2002) Evidence-based practices in geriatric mental health care. *Psychiatric Services*, 53(11), 1419–1431.
12. Prince M, Knapp M, Guerchet M, et al. (2014) *Dementia UK*, 2nd edition. London: Alzheimer's Society

13. Carers UK. (2015). *State of caring 2015*. London: Carers UK. carersuk.org/for-professionals/policy/policy-library/state-of-caring-2015 [Accessed 21/03/2023].

14. *Royal College of Psychiatry: Guidance for Commissioners of Older People's Mental Health Services*. National Collaborating Centre for Mental Health. (2021). *The framework for community mental health for adults and older adults: Support, care and treatment*. Part 1. London: National Collaborating Centre for Mental Health.

15. Samudra N, Patel N, Womack KB, Khemani P, Chitnis S (2016). Psychosis in Parkinson disease: A review of etiology, phenomenology, and management. *Drugs & Aging*, 33, 855–863.

16. Zhang JF, Wang XX, Feng Y, Fekete R, Jankovic J, Wu YC (2021). Impulse control disorders in Parkinson's disease: Epidemiology, pathogenesis and therapeutic strategies. *Frontiers in Psychiatry*, 12, 635494.

17. Rolinski M, Szewczyk-Krolikowski K, Tomlinson PR, et al. (2014) REM sleep behaviour disorder is associated with worse quality of life and other non-motor features in early Parkinson's disease. *Journal of Neurology, Neurosurgery & Psychiatry*, 85, 560–566.

18. Livingston G, Huntley J, Sommerlad A, Ames D, Ballard C, Banerjee S, Brayne C, Burns A, Cohen-Mansfield J, Cooper C, Costafreda SG (2020). Dementia prevention, intervention, and care: 2020 report of the Lancet Commission. *The Lancet*, 396(10248), 413–446.

19. Turner J, Kelly B (2000). Emotional dimensions of chronic disease. *Western Journal of Medicine*, 172(2), 124.

20. Lane CA, Hardy J, Schott JM (2018). Alzheimer's disease. *European Journal of Neurology*, 25(1), 59–70.

21. Korczyn AD, Vakhapova V, Grinberg LT (2012). Vascular dementia. *Journal of the Neurological Sciences*, 322(1–2), 2–10.

22. McKeith IG, Boeve BF, Dickson DW, Halliday G, Taylor JP, Weintraub D, Aarsland D, Galvin J, Attems J, Ballard CG, Bayston A (2017). Diagnosis and management of dementia with Lewy bodies: Fourth consensus report of the DLB Consortium. *Neurology*, 89(1), 88–100.

23. Wilson JE, Mart MF, Cunningham C, Shehabi Y, Girard TD, MacLullich AM, Slooter AJ, Ely EW (2020). Delirium. *Nature Reviews Disease Primers*, 6(1), 90.

24. Evans M, Mottram P (2000). Diagnosis of depression in elderly patients. *Advances in Psychiatric Treatment*, 6(1), 49–56.

25. Cleare A, Pariante CM, Young AH, Anderson IM, Christmas D, Cowen PJ, Dickens C, Ferrier IN, Geddes J, Gilbody S, Haddad PM (2015). Evidence-based guidelines for treating depressive disorders with antidepressants: A revision of the 2008 British Association for Psychopharmacology guidelines. *Journal of Psychopharmacology*, 29(5), 459–525.

26. Depp CA, Lindamer LA, Folsom DP, Gilmer T, Hough RL, Garcia P, et al. (2005). Differences in clinical features and mental health service use in bipolar disorder across the lifespan. *American Journal of Geriatric Psychiatry*, 13(4), 290–298.

27. Nebhinani N, Pareek V, Grover S (2014). Late-life psychosis: An overview. *Journal of Geriatric Mental Health*, 1(2), 60.

28. Wolitzky-Taylor KB, Castriotta N, Lenze EJ, Stanley MA, Craske MG (2010). Anxiety disorders in older adults: A comprehensive review. *Depression and Anxiety*, 27(2), 190–211.

29. McGrath A, Crome P, Crome IB (2005). Substance misuse in the older population. *Postgraduate Medical Journal*, 81(954), 228–231.

30. Conwell Y, Van Orden K, Caine ED (2011). Suicide in older adults. *Psychiatric Clinics*, 34(2), 451–468.

31. Penders KA, Peeters IG, Metsemakers JF, Van Alphen SP (2020). Personality disorders in older adults: A review of epidemiology, assessment, and treatment. *Current Psychiatry Reports*, 22, 1–14.
32. Shear MK, Ghesquiere A, Glickman K (2013). Bereavement and complicated grief. *Current Psychiatry Reports*, 15, 1–7.
33. Shear MK, Mulhare E (2008). Complicated grief. *Psychiatric Annals*, 38(10).

5   Psychotherapy

Arun Arujun Bhaskaran

The Royal College of Psychiatrists expects trainees to have a sound working knowledge of different psychological interventions in order to make appropriate referrals and provide psychoeducation to their patients.

Effectiveness of psychotherapy

- According to the American Psychiatric Association, about **75%** of people who enter therapy show benefit from it.

  - Benefits include **symptom relief, improved social functioning,** fewer **sick days** and **increased job satisfaction.**[1]

- Benefits **persist** when therapy ends and last longer than the effects of some non-psychological interventions.
- When combined with **pharmacotherapy**, improved outcomes in **depression, social phobia, panic disorder** and **bulimia** and equivocal outcomes in **schizophrenia** and **dysthymia** are observed.

  - Found to **hasten recovery, reduce relapse, improve medication compliance** and **reduce long-term healthcare costs.**[2]

- **Therapeutic alliance** is the single best predictor of outcome.
- Evidence for different psychological interventions is restricted due to **meta-analyses** missing declarations of interest, studies with **smaller sample sizes, difficulties** in **defining outcomes**, lack of **appropriate placebos** and **non-specific** and **pragmatic** factors.[3]

Principles and techniques of psychosocial therapies

Dynamic psychotherapy[4-7]

Underlying principles:

- Psychopathology stems from **childhood experiences**.

DOI: 10.4324/9781003376163-5

- **Repressed** memories of these experiences form the **unconscious mind**.
- Unconscious processes influence past, current and future events and relationships (**psychic determinism**).
- **Ego defence mechanisms** shield the unconscious.

Aims of psychotherapy:

- A **therapeutic alliance** enables a patient to trust and confide in their therapist.
  - **Interpretation** of the therapeutic alliance helps the therapist understand early relationships.
  - Therapists consider how patients feel and act towards them (**transference**) and how they feel about the patient (**counter-transference**).
- **Free association** and **dream analysis** help uncover unconscious processes.
- Therapists consider barriers like **ego defence mechanisms** and bring them to the **conscious** (see graphic).
  - Once barriers have surfaced, therapists and patients '**work through**' and develop new ways of coping.

Practicalities:

- Usually **long-term** over months and years.
  - **Brief psychotherapy** can be done on a time-limited basis with clear demarcated goals.
- Occurs on a **regular basis** (usually weekly).
- Can be **analytical** or **supportive** in nature.
- Wide range of **clinical indications** including depression, anxiety and anorexia.
- Contraindications include:
  - *Absence of psychological mindedness*
  - *Limited resilience and 'weak ego strength'*
  - *Acute psychosis*
  - *Active heavy substance misuse*
  - *Active severe suicidal thoughts/self-harm*
- Side effects include **negative therapeutic reactions** or **termination reactions**.
  - Uncovering the unconscious can be destabilising and patients may have a '**repetition compulsion**' (actively re-enacting past behaviours).

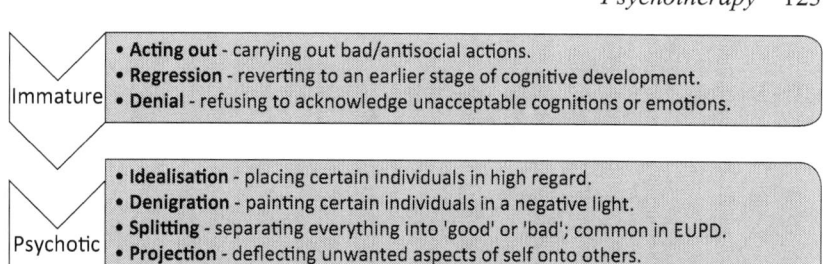

Immature
- **Acting out** - carrying out bad/antisocial actions.
- **Regression** - reverting to an earlier stage of cognitive development.
- **Denial** - refusing to acknowledge unacceptable cognitions or emotions.

Psychotic
- **Idealisation** - placing certain individuals in high regard.
- **Denigration** - painting certain individuals in a negative light.
- **Splitting** - separating everything into 'good' or 'bad'; common in EUPD.
- **Projection** - deflecting unwanted aspects of self onto others.
- **Projective identification** - projected ideas are assimilated by others.

Neurotic
- **Repression** - certain thoughts and feelings are held in the unconscious.
- **Intellectualisation** - negative thoughts or feelings are considered and explained in non-emotional ways.
- **Rationalisation** - negative thoughts or feelings are justified.
- **Reaction formation** - expressed thoughts and feelings are the polar opposite to what is truly felt or believed.
- **Magical thinking** - performing certain actions are believed to stop certain things happening; common in OCD.
- **Displacement** - negative thoughts and feelings are directed away from the source.

Mature
- **Sublimation** - use of adaptive coping mechanisms to deal with unacceptable thoughts and feelings.
- **Humour** - use of comedy to manage unacceptable thoughts.
- **Altruism** - diverting negative energy into positive actions.

Figure 5.1 Ego defence mechanisms

Key players[8]

Table 5.1 Important figures in the field of psychodynamic psychotherapy

Joseph Breuer	• Freud's mentor, inspired a lot of his works.
	• His 'Studies on Hysteria' (1895) examined the long-term impact of 'psychic trauma'.
Sigmund Freud	• Considered the 'father' of psychoanalysis.
	• Used 'Models of the Mind' to explain the mind's working.
	• *Topographical – unconscious, preconscious and conscious*
	•˙ *Structural – id, ego, superego*
	• Argued sexual desire was an individual's life force (eros).
	• *Suggested 4 psychosexual stages (oral, anal, phallic and genital) and the Oedipus/Electra complexes ('penis envy')*
	• Also coined the term 'Thanatos' (one's death instinct).
	• Freud's seminal work was 'The Interpretation of Dreams' (1900).
	• Described 'free association' as a strategy to overcome 'repressed' memories and reveal the unconscious.
	• *Dreams and parapraxes ('Freudian slips') provide other clues to the unconscious.*
	• Established the Vienna Psychoanalytic Society and later the International Psychoanalytic Association.

(Continued)

Table 5.1 (Continued)

Carl Jung	• Appointed by Freud as his successor to lead the International Psychoanalytic Association. • Worked with Freud on 'The Psychology of Dementia Praecox'. • Built on Freud's work and described the 'personal unconscious' and 'collective unconscious'. • Other Jungian concepts include: anima/animus, archetypes and extra/introversion.
Anna Freud	• Freud's daughter. • Published 'The Ego and the Mechanism of Defence' in 1936. • Did a lot of work on psychoanalysis in children.
Melanie Klein	• Highlighted children's play as a means to understand the workings of their minds. • Introduced the concepts of the paranoid-schizoid and depressive positions.
Donald Winicott	• Did a lot of work on children's development and parenting. • Concepts introduced included the importance of 'transitional objects' and the 'good enough mother' who 'holds'.
Wilfred Bion	• Build on the idea of holding and discussed professionals 'containing' individuals.
Other Neo-Freudians	• Generally agreed with Freud regarding early experiences and their impact on development but focused less on the sexual aspects and proposed other ideas: • *Alfred Adler – discussed the impact of feelings of inferiority on development and coined the term 'inferiority complex'* • *Erik Erickson – devised psychosocial stages of development and described crises at each life stage* • *Karen Horney – proposed 'womb envy' in women*

Family therapy[9–11]

* Roots in **general systems theory**.
* Informed by the field of **cybernetics**.
* Belief that individuals are a '**process of their relationships**' and shouldn't be considered in isolation.
* Therapists are **observers** of **systems**, but the lines are blurred between **observers** and the **observed**.

  * **Self-reflexivity** and **therapeutic curiosity** are important skills.

* **Genograms, family scripts** and **life cycles** are commonly used tools.
* Consideration is given to parenting, communication styles, life events, gender and cultural expectations.

Different models of family therapy[12]

Table 5.2 Different approaches to family therapy

Structural (Minuchin)	• Identifies and reconfigures family boundaries, hierarchies and subsystems. • Techniques include family mapping, re-enactments and reframing.

Strategic (Haley)	• Considers the function of problem behaviours in maintaining homeostasis. • Techniques include paradoxical injunction, restraining and metaphors.
Systemic (Milan)	• Focuses on interactions between family members. • Techniques include circular questioning and hypothesising.
Others	• Narrative. • Transgenerational. • Cognitive behavioural. • Solution-focused. • Psychoanalytical. • Psychoeducational.

Goals of treatment

In children and young people:

- Sleep, feeding and attachment in infancy.
- Child abuse and neglect.
- Conduct and behavioural difficulties, including attention and hyperactivity.
- Emotional difficulties (depression, anxiety, grief, suicidality).
- Physical health problems (enuresis, encopresis, recurrent abdominal pain, poorly controlled asthma and diabetes).
- Substance misuse.
- Eating disorders.

In adults:

- Relationship and psychosexual difficulties.
- Affective disorders (anxiety, depression).
- Substance misuse.
- Schizophrenia (particularly tackling issues of expressed emotion and providing psychoeducation).

Behavioural therapy

Functional analysis can be used to understand individuals' behaviours and help formulate treatment plans by assessing:

- **Antecedents** (what happens in the lead-up to the behaviour).
- **Behaviours** (what actions occur).
- **Consequences** (what occurs afterwards).[13]

Behavioural approaches[14–16]

Systematic desensitisation: used in anxiety disorders, based on the premise that feelings of anxiety and calm are mutually exclusive and inversely proportionate.

- A patient is given **relaxation training** and taught **autogenic strategies** (focusing on breath/different parts of the body), **mental imagery** and **progressive muscle relaxation**.
- Patient is exposed to an **anxiety-inducing situation** and encouraged to make use of the various relaxation techniques.

  - *The patient can devise a 'hierarchy' of fearful situations and be exposed to these in a step-wise fashion ('graded exposure')*
  - *The patient can be 'flooded' and exposed in real life to their biggest fear straight away*
  - *The patient can be encouraged to imagine their biggest fear in their mind ('implosion' or 'imaginal flooding')*

- Over time, **reciprocal inhibition** results in a reduction in anxiety symptoms.

Habit reversal training – patients with obsessive-compulsive disorder (**OCD**)/**tics** are given strategies to '**counteract**' **problematic behaviours**, i.e., if a patient has a tic which forces them to twist their neck to the right, they are encouraged to practice twisting their neck to the left.

Operant conditioning – use of reward (positive) or punishment (negative) **reinforcers** to increase or decrease certain behaviours, i.e., use of disulfiram in alcohol dependence or star charts in nocturnal enuresis.

Shaping and chaining – strategies to **reinforce** and **mould (shape)** or successively **build up (chain)** positive behaviours over time, i.e., rewarding an individual with a significant learning disability for notifying a caregiver when they need the toilet, then to going to the bathroom and successfully using the toilet to attend to their self-care.

Cue-exposure – considering **antecedents** in the lead-up to behaviour and controlling for these, i.e., if loud environments precipitate emotional outbursts in a child with autism spectrum disorder (ASD), pre-empting this and providing ear defenders when going to a shopping centre.

Habituation – **repeated exposure** to a feared stimulus over time can reduce anxiety, i.e., a child who is worried about attending school can be encouraged to visit the school playground, then the classroom and slowly build up more and more time there.

Social skills training – can be used in a variety of long-term conditions, i.e., schizophrenia or autism, for example to **aid social impairments**. Modelling and role-play can have a role, as well as functional skills, i.e., self-care, communicating with others.

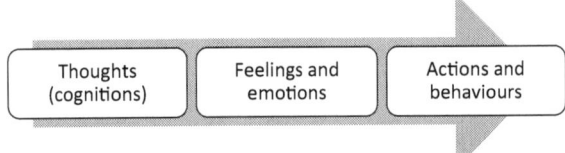

Figure 5.2 Aaron Beck's cognitive model for non-psychotic disorders

Cognitive therapy

Aaron Beck's cognitive model for non-psychotic disorders[17]:

Targeting unhelpful cognitions can impact associated behaviour[18–20]:

1. **Schemas** (negative core beliefs), i.e., 'I am no good'.
2. **Negative automatic thoughts** (reflex cognitions to a situation), i.e., 'There is no way I am going to pass this exam'.
3. **Maladaptive cognitive assumptions** (can be remembered using the mnemonic COMMS-PAD):

Table 5.3 Maladaptive cognitive assumptions

Assumption	Definition	Example
Catastrophising	Assuming the worst possible outcome.	'I failed my A-levels, now I will never get into university and my life is over'.
Over-generalising	Assuming the same outcome for everything.	After a date fails to text you back, thinking 'No one will be interested in me'.
Magnification	Giving undue weight to 1 aspect of a situation.	'I won't get the job because I forgot to shake the interviewer's hand'.
Minimisation	Downplaying or dismissing a positive outcome.	'I only passed the exam because the benchmark was so low'.
Selective abstraction	Focusing on a single negative outcome.	After failing Paper B, assuming you will never get your MRCPsych despite passing Paper A with flying colours.
Personalisation	Attributing all blame for negative outcomes to oneself.	'I lost the football match for the team because I didn't score that penalty at the end'.
Arbitrary inference	'Magical thinking'	'I'm not going to pass my theory test again because it's on a Wednesday again'.
Dichotomous thinking	'Black or white'/ 'all or nothing' thinking	'Getting this promotion is the only thing that will progress my career, if I don't get it my career is over'.

Ways to target unhelpful cognitions[21,22]:

- **Guided discovery** helps patients identify cognitions.
  - **Self-monitoring** through journals is encouraged.

- **Behavioural experiments** (such as **exposure-response prevention** in OCD and **selective physical attention** in health anxiety) can help patients challenge and shift cognitions.
- **Thought stopping/postponement** can be employed.
- **Ruminating** on negative thoughts can lead to **avoidance** and **safety behaviours**, perpetuating difficulties. Methods to **stop rumination**, safety behaviours and avoidance can therefore be helpful.

Cognitive model for psychotic disorders[23]:

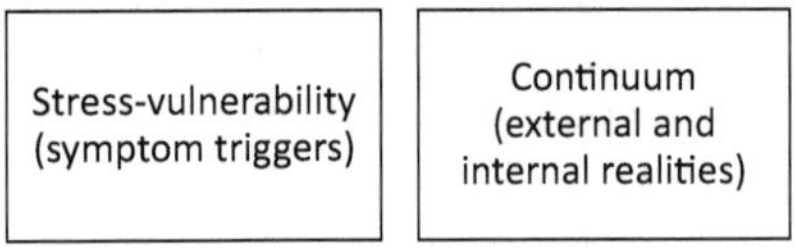

Stress-vulnerability (symptom triggers)	Continuum (external and internal realities)

Figure 5.3 Cognitive model for psychotic disorders

Techniques employed include:

- **Coping strategy enhancement** through sleep hygiene, relaxation training.
- **Relapse** indicator **identification** and **control**.
- **Graded reality testing** utilising **inference chaining** and **peripheral questioning**.

Group therapy

Historical roots of group therapy[24]

- Pioneered by **Pratt** in 1905 – held '**general-care instruction classes**' for discharged tuberculosis (TB) patients emotionally impacted by the disease.
- **Burrow** experimented with group therapy techniques in 1925 following frustrations with individual psychoanalysis.

  - *Hoped to change the **authoritarian** position of the therapist and consider **interpersonal relationships** more*

- **Schilder** and **Wender** used group therapy in prisoners and patients discharged from psychiatric hospitals in the 1930s.

  - *Increasing interest in group therapy for individuals under age 18 in this period*

- **World War II** saw a massive increase in group techniques owing to the large numbers of soldiers requiring intervention.

Group processes[25,26]

Before **formation** of the group. therapists should consider:

- Patients' life states.
- Patients' diagnoses.
- Patients' level of social functioning.
- Patients' proposed treatment plans.

Stages of the group formation include:

1. **Trust phase** – set-up of a safe and contained environment.
2. **Differentiation phase** – individuals start opening up and 'being themselves'.
3. **Working phase** – individuals make use of knowledge and skills they learn.
4. **Termination phase** – individuals separating and processing endings.

Different **group therapeutic factors** include[27-29]:

Table 5.4 Group therapeutic factors

Bion's 'basic assumptions' (states when groups derail)	Foulkes matrices	Yalom's 'curative factors' for effective therapy
• Dependency. • Pairing. • Fight–flight.	• Foundation matrix – commonalities needed between members for a group to be successful. • Dynamic matrix – changing dynamics and interactions between members through mirroring, exchange, free floating discussion, resonance and translation.	• Universality. • Group cohesiveness. • Altruism. • Instillation of hope. • Imparting of information. • Interpersonal learning. • Development of socialising techniques. • Imitative behaviour. • Corrective recapitulation of the primary family group. • Catharsis. • Existential factors.

Different models of group therapy

- **Psychoanalytical/dynamic.**
- **Expressive therapies** – i.e., psychodrama, art and music therapy.
- **Cognitive behavioural groups.**
- **Support groups.**
- **Psychoeducational groups.**
- **Skills groups** – i.e., life skills groups for those with chronic mental illness, social skills training in ASD.

Other therapeutic models

Interpersonal therapy (IPT)[30]

Psychologists: Klermann, Weissman
Premise: symptoms reactive to relationship difficulties.
Characteristics: structured, time-limited (12–16 sessions), commonly 1-on-1, 'here and now'.
Techniques: role transitions, grief, interpersonal disputes and deficits.
Indications: depression, eating disorders.

Cognitive analytical therapy (CAT)[31]

Psychologists: Ryle
Premise: combines psychoanalytical and cognitive behavioural therapy (CBT) approaches in order to understand the root of cognitions that drive problematic behaviours.
Characteristics: time-limited (16–24 sessions divided into reformulation, recognition and revision phases), explores past experiences.
Techniques: procedural sequence models (traps, snags and dilemmas), restricted role repertoires, reciprocal-role templates for emotionally unstable personality disorder (EUPD) patients, goodbye letters.
Indications: depression, anxiety, personality disorders.

Dialectic Behaviour Therapy (DBT)[32]

Psychologists: Linehan
Premise: acceptance' (helping patients come to terms with who they are) and 'change' (encouraging them to replace harmful behaviours with more adaptive ones).
Characteristics: can be 121 or group.
Techniques: 4 'modules' (mindfulness, improving interpersonal effectiveness, distress tolerance, emotional regulation).
Indications: EUPD, particularly self-harm and recurrent suicide attempts.

Gestalt therapy[33]

Psychologists: Perls, Goodman
Premise: humanistic approach focusing on self-awareness and barriers to this; empowers patients to respond differently (experiential freedom) in situations and take responsibility for their actions.
Characteristics: major focus on 'here and now', 121 commonly.
Techniques: empty chair, role plays and re-enactments, exaggeration exercises, dream work, dialogue.
Indications: anxiety, depression.

Client centred therapy[34]

Psychologists: Rogers
Premise: form of 'humanistic counselling'; belief that patients have the intrinsic ability to change and should direct this change themselves.
Characteristics: non-directive, 121 commonly.
Techniques: unconditional positive regard, self-concept.
Indications: relationship difficulties, low self-esteem, stress and anxiety management.

Transactional analysis[35]

Psychologists: Berne
Premise: analysing social interactions can determine the 'ego state' of patients and subsequently help understand certain actions and behaviours.
Characteristics: 121 or group setting (including family or couples).
Techniques: parent-adult-child models, unconscious scripts, strokes, redecision, recovery of spontaneity, awareness and intimacy.
Indications: relationship difficulties, anger issues, low self-esteem.

Mentalisation-based therapy[36]

Psychologists: Bateman, Fonagy
Premise: based on attachment theory; aims to increase awareness of self and others' emotional states and to validate.
Characteristics: treatment can last 12–18 months.
Techniques: 'transitional area of relatedness', 'minor interpretations'.
Indications: EUPD (borderline subtype).

References

1. Psychiatry.org. What is psychotherapy? Accessed 03/23
2. https://evidence.nihr.ac.uk/alert/combined-drug-and-psychological-therapies-may-be-most-effective-for-depression/ Accessed 03/23
3. Asen, E. (2002) Outcome research in family therapy. *Advances in Psychiatric Treatment* 8, 230–238
4. Bateman, A., Brown, D., and Pedder, J. (2010) *Introduction to psychotherapy*, 4th edition. New York: Routledge
5. www.bacp.co.uk/about-therapy/types-of-therapy/psychodynamic-therapy/ Accessed 03/23
6. www.foundationforchange.org.uk/ego-defence-mechanisms-handout Accessed 03/23
7. Bateman, A., and Holmes, J. (1995) *Introduction to psychoanalysis: Contemporary theory and practice*. London: Routledge.
8. Wright, P., Stern, J., and Phelan, M. (2012) *Core psychiatry*, 3rd edition. London: Saunders Elsevier.
9. Carter, E., and McGoldrick, M. (1984). *The family life cycle*. New York: Gardiner Press.
10. www.aft.org.uk/page/whatisfamilytherapy Accessed 03/23

11. https://tavistockandportman.nhs.uk/care-andtreatment/treatments/family-therapy/ Accessed 03/23
12. www.regain.us/advice/family/family-therapy-theories-modalities-and-efficacy/ Accessed 03/23
13. Dyer, K. (2013) Antecedent-behavior-consequence (A-B-C) analysis. In Volkmar, F. R. (eds), *Encyclopedia of autism spectrum disorders*. New York: Springer. https://doi.org/10.1007/978-1-4419-1698-3_1003
14. Pyles, D. A. M., and Baily, J. S. (1990) Diagnosing severe behavior problems. In Repp, A. C., and Singh, N. N. (eds.), *Perspectives on the use of aversive and nonaversive interventions for persons with developmental disabilities* (pp. 381–401). London: Sycamore Publishing Company.
15. Feldman, M. A., and Griffiths, D. (1997) Comprehensive assessment of severe behavior problems. In Singh, N. N. (ed.), *Prevention and treatment of severe behavior problems: Models and methods in developmental disabilities*. Pacific Grove, CA; Sycamore, IL: Brookes Publishing Company and Sycamore Publishing.
16. Hanley, G. P., et al. (2003) Functional analysis of problem behavior: A review. *Journal of Applied Behavior Analysis* 36, 147–185
17. Beck, J. S. (2011) *Cognitive behavior therapy: Basics and beyond*, 2nd edition. New York: The Guilford Press.
18. Morris, E., and Oliver, J. (2012) *In cognitive behaviour therapies*, ed. Dryden. Thousands Oaks: SAGE Publications.
19. Padesky, C. A. (1994) Schema change processes in cognitive therapy. *Clinical Psychology & Psychotherapy* 1, 267–278
20. Clark, D. A., and Beck, A. T. (1999) *Scientific foundations of cognitive theory and therapy of depression*. New York: Wiley.
21. Chambless, D. L., and Gillis, M. M. (1993) Cognitive therapy of anxiety disorders. *Journal of Consulting and Clinical Psychology* 61, 248–260.
22. Bennett-Levy, J., Butler, G., Fennel, M., et al. (2004) *Oxford guide to behavioural experiments in cognitive therapy*. Oxford: Oxford University Press.
23. Kingdon, D. G., and Turkington, D. (1994) *Cognitive behaviour therapy of schizophrenia*. Hove: Lawrence Earlbaum.
24. Bechelli, L. P., and dos Santos, M. A. (2004) Psicoterapia de grupo: como surgiu e evoluiu [Group psychotherapy: how it emerged and evolved]. *Rev Lat Am Enfermagem* 12(2), 242–249. Portuguese. Doi: 10.1590/s0104-11692004000200014.
25. Stangor, C. Group processes. *Oxford Research Encyclopedia of Psychology*. https://oxfordre.com/psychology/view/10.1093/acrefore/9780190236557.001.0001/acrefore-9780190236557-e-255 Accessed 21/04/23
26. www.apa.org/topics/psychotherapy/group-therapy Accessed 03/23
27. Sigmind, K., Folmo, E., et al. (2019) *Personality and the group matrix*. London: Group Analysis, pp. 503–519.
28. Bion, W. Group dynamics – The "basic assumptions". *Technology Trends*, primidi. com Accessed 03/23
29. Yalom, I. D. (1985) *The theory and practice of group psychotherapy*, 3rd edition. London: Basic Books.
30. www.counselling-directory.org.uk/interpersonal-therapy.html Accessed 03/23
31. Denman, C. (2001) Cognitive analytical therapy. *Advances in Psychiatric Treatment* 7, 243–252
32. www.mind.org.uk/information-support/drugs-and-treatments/talking-therapy-and-counselling/dialectical-behaviour-therapy-dbt/ Accessed 03/23
33. www.bacp.co.uk/about-therapy/types-of-therapy/gestalt/ Accessed 03/23
34. www.goodtherapy.org/learn-about-therapy/types/person-centered Accessed 03/23
35. https://patient.info/news-and-features/what-is-transactional-analysis-therapy Accessed 03/23
36. Fonagy, P., and Bateman, A. W. (2006) Mechanisms of change in mentalization-based treatment of BPD. *Journal of Clinical Psychology* 62(4), 411–430.

6   Child and adolescent psychiatry

Arun Arujun Bhaskaran

Children's rights and welfare[1]

- In **England**, a child is defined as '**anyone who has not yet reached their 18th birthday**'.
- **Northern Ireland** and Wales define a child as someone '**under the age of 18**'.
- In **Scotland**, the definition **changes** in different legal situations.

Laws governing the rights of children[1]

International:

- **UN Convention on the Rights of the Child** describes the right of every child to 'survive, grow, participate and fulfil their potential'.
- **European Convention on Human Rights** sets out a child's 'right to life, to be kept safe from torture and cruel treatment' and the 'right to an education', amongst others.

UK:

- **The Human Rights Act 1998**
- **The Equality Act 2010**

Safeguarding refers to the steps taken to ensure a child's wellbeing and protection from harm. **Child protection** is part of this process and involves identifying those suffering from or at significant risk of harm.

Following a series of high-profile abuse cases, the **1989 Children Act** placed new responsibilities on **local authorities** to provide help to vulnerable children and their families.[2,3]

Concepts covered in the act include[2,3]:

1. Shifts from **parental rights** *over* a child to **parental responsibility (PR)** *towards* a child.

   - **All mothers** gain PR upon birth of their child, as do fathers in **married couples**.

DOI: 10.4324/9781003376163-6

2. The value of **keeping families together**.
3. Identifying and providing help to **children in need**.
4. Provision of **housing** and **care** to those who have nobody with PR to care for them (**looked-after children**) and supporting them when **leaving care**.
5. Conducting **investigations** to determine whether a child is suffering from or likely to come to significant harm (including **Section 47 investigations**).
6. Assessing and reviewing the need for **supervision, interim care** and **emergency protection orders**.

Harm can stem from **adverse childhood experiences** such as abuse, neglect and household challenges (mental illness, substance misuse, domestic abuse).[4]

Note: children are now also considered victims of domestic abuse alongside affected partners.

Child protection[4,5]

Abuse is the **maltreatment** or **exploitation** of a person and can be **intentional harm** or the **failure** to **prevent** it.

Risk factors for abuse include:

- Socioeconomic deprivation.
- Parental mental illness and/or substance misuse.
- Parental experience of abuse or neglect as children.
- Children with learning disability (LD) or chronic physical health problems.[6]

Table 6.1 Different categories of abuse

Category of abuse	Definition	Signs and symptoms
Physical[7]	Intentional injury via any means.	• Recurrent unexplained injuries or marks. • Injuries with inconsistent narratives. • Failure to seek prompt medical attention for injuries.
Emotional/ psychological[7]	Making a young person feel worthless, unwanted or unloved.	• Low self-esteem and self-worth. • Self-harming behaviours.
Sexual[7]	Sexual activity between a child and an adult or non-consensual sexual activity between children.	• Sleep disturbance. • Sexual behaviour not in keeping with age/development. • Overfamiliarity or wariness of adults. • Injuries to genitals. • Urinary tract, vaginal or sexually transmitted infections. • Pregnancy.

Neglect[7]	Failure to adequately meet the needs of a child.	• Poor hygiene. • Hunger/thirst. • Failure to attend medical appointments. • School absence.
Fabricated (induced illness)[7]	Caregiver attempts to convince professionals that their child is ill/their illness is more serious than it actually is.	• Repeated presentations to medical professionals. • Exaggeration or lies about health. • Deliberate induction of symptoms, i.e., through poisoning. • Manipulation of test results.
Female genital mutilation (FGM)[8]	Procedure where female genitalia are cut, injured or changed without medical indication.	• Commonly presents to general practitioners (GPs) and obstetricians. • Travel to a country with high prevalence rates or missing education.

It is the duty of all professionals to safeguard young people and raise concerns regarding suspected suffering, abuse or neglect. It is a duty to discuss with line managers and safeguarding officers/leads and to promptly tell an appropriate agency.

Child and adolescent mental health services (CAMHS)[9–16]

Organised into 4 tiers[14]:

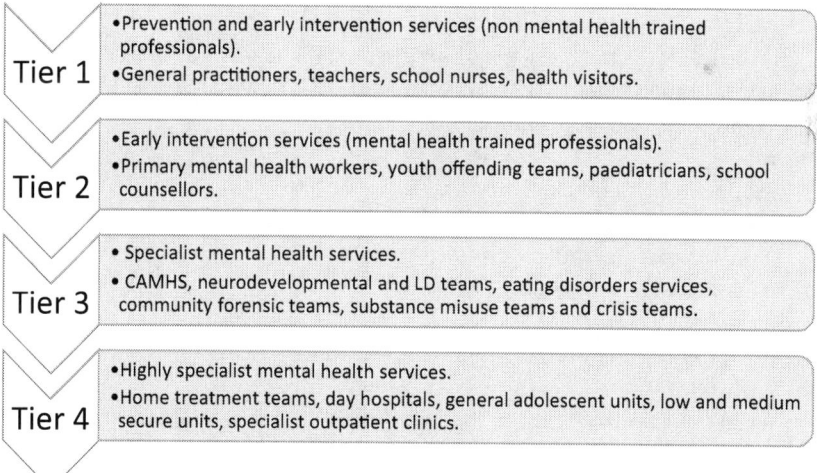

Tier 1
• Prevention and early intervention services (non mental health trained professionals).
• General practitioners, teachers, school nurses, health visitors.

Tier 2
• Early intervention services (mental health trained professionals).
• Primary mental health workers, youth offending teams, paediatricians, school counsellors.

Tier 3
• Specialist mental health services.
• CAMHS, neurodevelopmental and LD teams, eating disorders services, community forensic teams, substance misuse teams and crisis teams.

Tier 4
• Highly specialist mental health services.
• Home treatment teams, day hospitals, general adolescent units, low and medium secure units, specialist outpatient clinics.

Figure 6.1 Mental health support for young people in the UK

Source: Tier 4 services are provided on a regional/supra-regional basis and are commissioned nationally.

Focus of Tier 3 and 4 services on **multidisciplinary working**. Professionals involved include:

- Psychiatrists.
- Psychologists and psychotherapists.
- Therapists (art, play, drama) and counsellors.
- Paediatricians.
- Social workers.
- Support and youth workers.

Referrals to CAMHS can be made by **patients**, their **families** or **professionals** (GPs, paediatricians, nurses, teachers, social workers, youth workers, etc.).

In England, no national standards on waiting times exist apart from:

- **2 weeks** for patients with **psychosis**.
- **1 week** for patients with an **eating disorder** and urgent concerns.

All CAMHS services are under pressure and impacted by **chronic underinvestment** and **increasing demand** – the 'Cinderella of Cinderella services'.

The Children and Young People's Mental Health and Wellbeing Taskforce's **'The Future in Mind' (2015)** and the Children's Commissioner's **'Lightning Review' (2016)** emphasised the need to address the **challenges faced by CAMHS** and **inequalities in services**.

Reports highlighted concerns of **inappropriate hospital admissions** due to **inadequate community services**.

Inappropriate inpatient admission:

- **Separates** children and families.
- **Disrupts** social life and schooling.
- Adds to parental **guilt**.
- Can potentially be **stigmatising**.

Hersov (1994)[17] proposed the following indications for inpatient admissions:

- **Assessment** that cannot be completed to a good standard in the community.
- **Severe acute mental illness** needing multidisciplinary treatment team (MDT) input in a safe and contained environment.
- **Impaired physical states** requiring specialist input.
- **Adverse environmental circumstances** impacting recovery, including **gross overprotection**.

Mental, behavioural and developmental disorders in childhood[18-20]

A. Attachment disorders

Set of conditions in which sufferers struggle to forge meaningful emotional connections with others.

Prevalence

- The National Institute of Clinical Excellence (NICE) suggests that prevalence in the general population is *not well established*, but likely to be low.
- 2.5–20% of looked-after children estimated as having an attachment disorder.

Aetiology

Risk factors include:

- Looked-after children (care institutions, frequent moves between caregivers).
- Children separated from their parents due to illness, death, war, natural disasters, etc.
- Victims of abuse and/or neglect.

Presentation

2 main types of attachment disorder outlined in DSM-5:

- **Reactive attachment disorder (RAD)** – aloof and withdrawn from others; minimally seeks comfort or is comforted by adult caregivers. Can be associated with episodes of aggression and anxiety.
- **Disinhibited social engagement disorder (DSED)** – overly familiar and socially inappropriate with others.

Symptoms should be present at <5 years old.

Treatment

- Securing a loving and stable long-term placement for the child.
- Parent/caregiver support and training.
- Involvement of appropriate external agencies including social services.
- Play therapy and other therapeutic modalities may have a role (behavioural, trauma-focused CBT).

Outcomes

- Preventable.
- Without treatment can lead to emotional and behavioural disturbances (including anxiety and depression), developmental delay and involvement with the criminal justice system.
- RAD settles quickly with appropriate treatment but DSED can persist.

B. Conduct disorders

Prevalence

- High prevalence rates (5.6% of 5–16-year-olds in England).
- Rates increase throughout childhood.
- Males > females.
- Increased in inner city areas and areas of high socioeconomic deprivation.
- Ethnic variability.

Aetiology

- Neuropsychological deficits.
- Brain injury.
- Autonomic under-arousal.
- Certain temperaments, low tolerance to frustration.
- Maternal smoking.
- Paternal criminality.
- Low socioeconomic status.
- Institutionalised care, looked-after children.
- Harsh parenting styles.
- Family discord.
- Academic underachievement.
- Social isolation and poor peer relationships.
- Adverse childhood experiences, including childhood abuse.

Presentation

- Repetitive dissocial, aggressive or defiant behaviours (violence and aggression towards people or animals, damage to property, fire setting with the intention to harm, deceit or theft)
- Enduring in nature (DSM specifies 12-month duration).
- Major violations of age-appropriate social expectations.
- Can be socialised (peer pressure, conformity) or unsocialised.
- Oppositional defiant disorder (ODD) describes a milder form without the major violations of social expectations and usually presents in younger children.

Treatment

- Exclude and treat psychiatric comorbidities, including ADHD.
- Risperidone is used for short-term management of aggressive behaviours.
- Psychoeducation and training/support for caregivers.
- Involvement of external agencies (social services, mentors, youth charities).
- Systemic therapies (multisystemic therapy, functional family therapy).

Outcomes

- Without intervention, can lead to dropping out of education, employment and relationship difficulties, vulnerabilities to gang-related activity, crime, substance misuse, unwanted sexually transmitted diseases and pregnancies.
- Can progress to antisocial personality disorder in adulthood.

C. Attention deficit hyperactivity disorder (ADHD)[21]

Prevalence

- Global prevalence estimated around 5%.

    - *In the USA, estimated to be up to 10%*

- Males > females.

Aetiology

- Strong genetic component – mean heritability of 76% in twin studies.
- Maternal smoking and low birth weight are the most strongly associated environmental factors.
- Other risk factors including:

    - *Alcohol and substance misuse (particularly heroin) during pregnancy*
    - *Foetal hypoxia and acquired brain injury*
    - *Epilepsy and certain genetic syndromes (Fragile X, velocardiofacial)*
    - *Lead poisoning*
    - *Institutionalised care, looked-after children*

Presentation

- Core symptoms of:

    - *Hyperactivity (excessive motor activity and difficulties sitting still)*
    - *Inattention (inability to focus on low-stimulus tasks that do not provide frequent rewards, easily distracted and disorganised)*

- *Impulsivity (tendency to do or say things without thoroughly assessing the consequences)*
- Should impact function.
- Present in multiple settings (school, home, public).
- Symptoms usually evident prior to age 12 but can present later.

  - *Older diagnostic manuals specified prior to the age of 7*

- The Connor's questionnaire can be a useful screening/diagnostic tool.

Treatment

- ADHD-focused group/individual parent-training programmes.
- Psychoeducation for parents/caregivers and schools.
- CBT (particularly focusing on social skills, self-control and active listening).
- Medications:

  - *Not routinely offered to children <5 years of age*
  - *Methylphenidate is usually the first line, switching to lisdexamfetamine if 6-week trial proves ineffective*
  - *Immediate release preparations should be avoided if there is a risk of misuse or diversion*
  - *Modified-release preparations enable once daily dosages and reduce stigma but immediate release enable flexibility*
  - *Monitor heart rate, blood pressure, height and weight closely*
  - *Consider an electrocardiogram (ECG) and cardiology opinion for cardiac symptoms, history of congenital heart disease or sudden death in a first-degree relative <40 years*
  - *Consider atomoxetine or guanfacine if stimulants are intolerable/not effective*
  - *Monitor for liver dysfunction and suicidal thoughts with atomoxetine*
  - *Clonidine can be considered in cases of worsening tics on other medications*

Outcomes

- Meta-analyses of cohort studies found that by mid-20s, 15% of patients were in complete remission, 65% were in partial remission and 15% retained the full diagnosis.

  - *Inattention endured with time whereas hyperactivity and impulsivity improved*

- Untreated, ADHD can impact schooling, academic performance, peer relations and self-esteem.

  - *It can also lead to conduct disorder and associated complications*

D. Anxiety disorders

Table 6.2 Types of anxiety disorders in childhood and adolescence

Separation anxiety disorder (SAD)	• Most common anxiety-related disorder in children. • Prevalence estimated 1–4%. • Typical onset in early childhood. • Risk factors include: parental loss, extended parental absences, looked-after children and parental alcohol misuse. • Presents as recurrent and excessive emotional distress anticipating or being away from home or caregivers. • *Should be present for at least 4 weeks, be disproportionate to age and development and impact function* • Treatment can include selective serotonin reuptake inhibitors (SSRIs) and CBT. • Can progress to agoraphobia +/- panic disorder if untreated.
School refusal	• Prevalence unknown. • Classically presents gradually at transition points (i.e., primary to secondary school) or suddenly following school holidays. • Considered a symptom rather than a diagnosis – exact aetiology should be determined (separation anxiety, bullying/exam pressures, conduct disorder, depression, etc.). • Treatment dependent on cause. • Quick identification and reintegration improve prognosis.

Selective mutism	• Rare – prevalence estimated 0.7%.
	• Females > males.
	• Typical onset in early childhood.
	• Risk factors include family history of selective mutism or anxiety disorders and past trauma.
	• Presents as an inability to speak in certain settings, i.e., at school, over 1–2 months.
	  • *Ability to speak without restriction in places they feel at ease, i.e., home*
	• Behavioural therapies including shaping, stimulus-fading and graded exposure are mainstay.
	  • *Speech and language input may play a role*
	• Untreated, can persist into adulthood and significantly impair functioning.

(Continued)

Table 6.2 (Continued)

Post-traumatic stress disorder (PTSD)	• Prevalence 10% in individuals <18 years old. • Estimated 30% of young people exposed to a potentially traumatic event develop PTSD symptoms. • Females > males. • Common precipitants include abuse, violent crimes, natural disasters and war. • Same symptoms as adult population. 　• *Regression, separation anxiety, somatisation, challenging behaviours, agitation and hyperactivity may also occur* 　• *Complex PTSD (c-PTSD) is seen in individuals with recurring or long-term exposure to traumatic events and can present with emotional dysregulation and difficulties with relationships* • Treatments can include trauma-focused CBT or EMDR (eye movement desensitisation and reprocessing). 　• *Medication should not routinely be prescribed unless comorbidities exist* • With appropriate treatment, full recovery can occur within 6 months, but risk of persistence and impairment exists without.
Obsessive-compulsive disorder (OCD)	• Rare – prevalence estimated 0.5%. • Pre-puberty, male preponderance, and from puberty onwards, more common in females. • Genetic predisposition, neuroanatomical and neurochemical changes have been implicated in research studies. 　• *Paediatric autoimmune neuropsychiatric disorders associated with Streptococcus (PANDAS) manifests as OCD symptomatology in young people following strep throat or scarlet fever* • Same symptoms as adults but tend to be secretive as self-conscious about compulsions. 　• Tic disorders, autism spectrum disorder (ASD) and other neurodevelopmental disorders are common comorbidities • NICE-recommended treatment options include: 　• *Guided self-help in cases of mild impairment* 　• *CBT (including exposure and response prevention) for moderate to severe cases* 　• *SSRIs if psychological interventions are ineffective or inappropriate* • Remission more likely in paediatric population than in adults – early intervention and before significant impact on functioning improved prognosis.
Specific phobias	• 3 years – animals. • 4–5 years – the dark. • 5 years – monsters and imaginary creatures. • Late childhood/early adolescence – open spaces. • Adolescence – illness and death, failure, sex. • Any age – storms and snakes.

E. Affective disorders[22–24]

Table 6.3 Types of affective disorders in childhood and adolescence

Depressive disorder	• WHO estimates 1.1% prevalence in 10–14-year-olds and 2.8% in 15–19-year-olds.
	  • *Rising incidence*
	• Post-puberty females > males.
	• 95% of major depression in young people associated with longstanding psychosocial difficulties.
	  • *Comorbidity is the rule!*
	• Diagnostic criteria same as in adults.
	  • *Full-blown depression rare pre-puberty but may present with irritability, somatic symptoms, school refusal and antisocial behaviour*
	  • *Anhedonia and social withdrawal are highly sensitive predictors*
	• Treatment options:
	  • *Conservative and guided self-help in mild cases*
	  • *Psychological interventions include CBT, IPT, family therapy and psychotherapy*
	  • *SSRIs are first line (fluoxetine, followed by sertraline or citalopram)*
	  • *The treatment for adolescents with depression study highlighted the better outcomes in combination treatment (psychological + pharmacological)*
	• Most affected recover within 2 years of onset but higher risk of relapse compared to adult counterparts.
	  • *'Scarring' from first episode may sensitise to further episodes*

Self-harm	• Very common and rising incidence. • *Completed suicide is the 3rd leading cause of adolescent mortality* • Deliberate self-harm higher in females, completed suicide higher in males. • Self-poisoning is the most common method.

Bipolar affective disorder	• 1% prevalence in adolescents.
	• Pre-puberty males > females, equal prevalence post puberty.
	• Family history, trauma and life events are observed risk factors.
	  • *Comorbid ADHD and substance misuse common*
	• For a diagnosis of bipolar, mania must be present with elated mood present on most days for most of the day in week prior.
	• Atypical antipsychotics are first line, followed by mood stabilisers if 2 different trials are unsuccessful.
	  • *Avoid valproate in females due to risk of teratogenicity and polycystic ovarian syndrome (PCOS)*
	  • *Higher doses of lithium may be required due to higher estimated glomerular filtration rate*
	• Early-onset bipolar disorder associated with chronicity, rapid cycling, treatment resistance and long-term functional decline.

F.   Psychosis

Prevalence

- Very early-onset schizophrenia (<13 years) is rare, but rates increase rarely in adolescence.
- Estimated that 20% of those with schizophrenia present with signs/symptoms before the age of 18.

Aetiology

- Genetic factors (first-degree relatives, twin studies).
- Neuroanatomical changes (enlarged lateral ventricles, reduced hippocampal volume).
- Dopamine imbalances.
- Cannabis misuse particularly in early adolescence (dose-response effect seen).
- Linked with physical health disorders, including infectious (malaria, human immunodeficiency virus [HIV], syphilis), autoimmune (anti-N-methyl-D-asparate receptor encephalitis) and metabolic (adrenocortical insufficiency).

Presentation

- Similar to adult population.
- Prodrome frequently seen.
- Hallucinations and negative symptoms common; catatonia less so.
- Psychotic symptoms not limited to schizophrenia in paediatric populations – consider affective disorders, substance misuse and ASD.

Treatment

- Medication algorithms similar to those for adults.
- Be wary of the increased sensitivity to side effects (extrapyramidal side effects, weight gain and metabolic effects, sedation, hyperprolactinaemia).
- Clozapine has a role in treatment resistance but causes increased susceptibility to neutropenia and seizures.
- Depots are not commonly used.
- Psychoeducation, family therapy and CBT have a role.

Outcomes

Earlier onset of schizophrenia tends to be more refractory to treatments and carry a poorer prognosis.

G. Eating disorders[25,26]

Prevalence

- Point prevalence estimated around 6.4% of the UK population.
- 25% of sufferers are male but frequently undiagnosed.
- Studies show a rising prevalence.
- Other specified feeding or eating disorder (OSFED) is the most common eating disorder following by binge eating disorder (BED).
- Anorexia nervosa and avoidant restrictive food intake disorder (ARFID) are the least prevalent.
- Onset typically in adolescence and early adulthood but can occur at any time.

Aetiology

Risk factors include:

- Positive family history (7–12% higher).
- Being overweight as a child.
- Perfectionistic traits, low self-esteem.
- Comorbid anxiety and depression.
- Professional/recreational pressures to be thin, i.e., dancing, modelling.
- Adverse childhood experiences.
- ASD and lifelong 'picky eaters' in ARFID.

Presentation

Table 6.4 Categories of eating disorder

Anorexia nervosa (AN)	• Weight loss and low body weight (BMI <17.5 or weight for height <85% expected). • Distorted body image and intense fear of weight gain. • Dietary restriction and/or compensatory behaviours (over-exercising, purging). • Loss of periods. • Physical complications including bradycardia, orthostatic hypotension, hypothermia, dry skin, hair loss, constipation and reduced muscle power.
Bulimia nervosa (BN)	• Weight usually within normal limits or above expected. • Bingeing episodes at least weekly over a period of 3 months followed by intense feelings of guilt and shame. • Compensatory behaviours to limit weight gain. • Physical symptoms including gastro-oesophageal reflux disease, bloating, feeling full and complications of self-induced vomiting (electrolyte disturbance, dental caries, Russell's sign and sore throat).

(Continued)

Table 6.4 (Continued)

Binge eating disorder (BED)	• Usually overweight or obese. • Bingeing episodes at least weekly over a period of 3 months without compensatory behaviours.
Avoidant/ restrictive food intake disorder (ARFID)	• Avoidance of specific foods or food groups. • Associated restriction in quantity of food consumed. • Not in keeping with religious or cultural norms or associated with a lack of food availability. • Can be due to sensory sensitivities, fear of negative consequences (feeling full, choking, vomiting) or a lack of interest in eating.
Other specified feeding or eating disorder (OSFED)	• Feeding or eating difficulties not meeting the thresholds for other diagnoses – may progress to anorexia/bulimia. • Preoccupation with food and distorted body image are usually present.

Treatment

- Medical Emergencies in eating disorders (MEED) guidelines from the Royal College of Psychiatrists can guide whether treatment can be undertaken in the community or if hospitalisation is required.
- Treatment of any physical health complications.
- Weight restoration with specialist dietician involvement.

  - *Caution with refeeding syndrome and shift to carbohydrate metabolism and insulin secretion causing intracellular electrolyte shifts*
  - *Resultant hypokalaemia, hypomagnesaemia, hypocalcaemia and hypophosphatemia can lead to arrhythmias, oedema, tetany, delirium and death*

- Harm minimisation from compensatory behaviours (avoidance of brushing teeth after vomiting, cessation of exercise, stopping laxatives).
- Psychoeducation for patients and caregivers.
- Medication options.

  - *No licensed treatments but olanzapine is used in AN and fluoxetine in BN*
  - *Treatment of psychiatric comorbidities particular depression and anxiety*

- Psychological treatments:

  - AN.

    - *Adults*
      - Cognitive behaviour therapy for eating disorders (CBT-ED)
      - Maudsley Model of Anorexia Nervosa Treatment for Adults (MANTRA)
      - Specialist supportive clinical management (SSCM)

- Focal psychodynamic therapy (FPT)
- *Children and young people*
  - Family therapy for anorexia nervosa (FT-AN)
  - CBT-ED
  - Adolescent-focused therapy for anorexia nervosa (AFP-AN)

- BN.

  - *Adults*
    - Guided self-help
    - CBT-ED
  - *Children and young people*
    - Family therapy for bulimia nervosa (FT-BN)
    - CBT-ED

- BED.
  - Guided self-help
  - Brief supportive sessions
  - Group/individual CBT-ED

Outcomes

- All eating disorders can persist if left untreated or treated inadequately.
- AN carries the highest rates of mortality through cardiac complications, infections and completed suicide.

  - *Positive prognosis in younger age group with shorter duration of illness – complete recovery less likely with increasing duration*

- BN associated with better recovery rates and lower mortality.
- More research is needed into the prognosis of the other eating disorders.

H. Autism spectrum disorders (ASD)[27]

Prevalence

- Worldwide, 1% of young people estimated to have ASD, but figures vary significantly and more research needed, especially in low income countries.

  - 700,000 children and adults in the UK living with ASD.

- Males:females (3:1–5:1).

Aetiology

- High heritability (70–90% concordance in monozygotic twins).
- Syndromic ASD associated with certain chromosomal abnormalities (seen in Rett, Fragile X and *MECP2* duplication syndromes).

- Congenital rubella infection.
- Valproate and SSRI use (conflicting data) during pregnancy.
- Parental age, maternal nutrition and exposure to mercury/lead has also been implicated.
- No causality between measles, mumps and rubella (MMR)/childhood vaccines and ASD.

Presentation

- Persistent impairment in social interaction and communication skills.

  - *Difficulties forming social relationships*
  - *Limited theory of mind and interest in others*
  - *Decreased early babble, delayed speech or mutism*
  - *Abnormalities in rhythm, intonation and pitch, echolalia, pronominal reversal and literal thinking*
  - *Difficulties understanding and using gestures and integrated verbal and non-verbal communications*

- Persistent restricted, repetitive and rigid patterns of behaviour, activities and interests.

  - *Circumscribed/unusual interests*
  - *Non-imaginative play*
  - *Insistence on sameness*

- Associated sensory hypo/hypersensitivities.
- Other signs and symptoms include motor stereotypies, hand flapping and other mannerisms, emotional outbursts and challenging behaviours.
- Rett syndrome characterised by normal early development followed by a partial or complete loss of skills.
- ICD-11 changes:

  - *Onset should occur during the 'developmental period'*
  - *Qualifies ASD with or without intellectual disability and with or without functional language impairments*
  - *Asperger's syndrome no longer a diagnosis in ICD-11*

Treatment

- Treatment of any comorbidities.
- Antipsychotics for behavioural management.
- Psychoeducation.
- Developing emotional and communication skills; life skills interventions.
- Functional assessments and behavioural therapies.
- Training and support for parents, caregivers and schools.

Outcomes

- Lifelong condition.

I.   Substance misuse[28]

- Latest figures show that cannabis is the most commonly misused substance in adolescence followed by alcohol.
- Nicotine, ecstasy and powder cocaine were also frequently used.
- Risk factors included comorbid mental illness, being a looked-after child and lack of education, employment or training.
- Number of young people taking up drugs and alcohol support has fallen each year since 2008.

J.   Tic disorders[29]

- Set of childhood onset neuropsychiatric disorders characterised by repetitive, abrupt and sudden non-rhythmic movements (grimacing, throat clearing, body writhing, throat clearing and blinking) or vocalisations (echolalia, coprolalia and palilalia).

Prevalence

- Relatively common neurodevelopmental disorder affecting 1% of the population.
- Males > females.

Aetiology

- Risk factors include positive family history, neuroanatomical changes (basal ganglia has been implicated) and neurochemical imbalances (particularly dopamine dysfunction).

Presentation

- Can be characterised by 1 or more vocal tics and/or 1 or more motor tics.

  - ***Tourette syndrome*** *characterised by both vocal and motor tics (most common subtype)*

- Can be *transient* (<12 months) or *chronic* (>12 months).
- ICD-11 categorises tics as *primary* or *secondary* to infection, drugs or illness.

Treatment

- Treat secondary causes and any comorbidities.

- Psychoeducation and psychological interventions are considered first-line treatments in the paediatric population.
  - *Habit reversal training (HRT)*
  - *Comprehensive behavioural intervention for tics (CBIT)*
  - *Exposure and response prevention (ERP)*
- Pharmacological treatment options: clonidine/guanfacine ◊ atypical antipsychotics (risperidone, aripiprazole) ◊ typical antipsychotics (haloperidol is the only licensed medication for Tourette syndrome).

Outcomes

Tends to improve and remit with age but may persist into adulthood.

K. Other childhood disorders

Table 6.5 Other mental health conditions in childhood and adolescence

Enuresis[30]	• 5–10% at 7 years, 1–2% in adolescents. • Repetitive voiding of urine into clothes or bed during the day or night beyond 5 years of age. • Primary or secondary (following period of acquired continence). • Not attributable to organic causes (medications, physical illness, etc.). • Behavioural interventions (alarms, reward charts) and desmopressin have a role in treatment. • Most cases resolve by adolescence but a small proportion persist into adulthood.
Encopresis[31,32]	• Less common than enuresis (1.6% of 10-year-olds). • Males > females. • Repetitive faecal soiling in inappropriate places (at least monthly over several months) beyond 4 years of age. • Constipation with overflow may or may not be present. • Can be primary or secondary and should not be attributable to organic disease. • Behavioural approaches. • Persistent with worsening of symptoms.
Pica	• Regular consumption of 'non-nutritive' substances beyond age 2 when individuals would be expected to distinguish between what is edible and what is not.
Gender incongruence	• Discrepancy between an individual's sex assigned at birth and their experienced gender; can occur in pre-pubertal children or adolescence and may be associated with a desire to transition via medical or surgical means.

References

1. Children and the Law. *NSPCC Learning*. https://learning.nspcc.org.uk/child-protection-system/children-the-law. Accessed 12/22.
2. Children Act 1989. What does it do?, Politics.co.uk. Accessed 12/22.
3. Children Act 1989. legislation.gov.uk. Accessed 12/22.
4. Child Protection and Safeguarding. *The Children's Society*, childrenssociety.org.uk Accessed 12/22.
5. Safeguarding Children and Child Protection. *NSPCC Learning*. https://learning.nspcc.org.uk/safeguarding-child-protection. Accessed 12/22.
6. Kessler, R. C., McLaughlin, K. A., Green, J. G., et al. Childhood adversities and adult psychopathology in the WHO. *World Mental Health Surveys. The British Journal of Psychiatry*. 2010;197(5):378–385. doi:10.1192/bjp.bp.110.080499.
7. Spotting the Signs of Child Abuse. *NSPCC* Accessed 12/22.
8. Female Genital Mutilation, who.int Accessed 12/22
9. NHS in England. A guide to mental health services in England. *A-Z NHS Choices*, 2016. www.nhs.uk/NHSEngland/AboutNHSservices/mental-health-services-explained/Pages/about-childrens-mental-health-services.aspx Accessed 12/22
10. CQC. Brief guide: Waiting times for community child and adolescent mental health services. *Care Quality Commission*, 2016. www.cqc.org.uk/sites/default/files/20170121_briefguide-camhs-waitingtimes.pdf, December 2016 Accessed 12/22
11. Children's Commissioner. Children's Commissioner's report lightning review: Access to child and adolescent mental health services, 2016. www.cqc.org.uk/sites/default/files/20170121_briefguide-camhs-waitingtimes.pdf Accessed 12/22
12. NHS England. Children and young people's mental health services baselining report local transformation plans review 2015, 2016. www.england.nhs.uk/mentalhealth/wp-content/uploads/sites/29/2015/08/nhse-camhs-baselining-summary1.pdf Accessed 12/22
13. NHS England. Child and adolescent mental health services (CAMHS) Tier 4 Report. *NHS England*, 2014. www.england.nhs.uk/wp-content/uploads/2014/07/camhs-tier-4-rep.pdf Accessed 12/22
14. www.hpftcamhs.nhs.uk/coming-to-camhs-what-to-expect/our-hpft-camhs-services/camhs-tiers/ Accessed 12/22
15. Frith E. CentreForum commission on children and young people's mental health: State of the nation. *CentreForum*, 2016. http://centreforum.org/live/wp-content/uploads/2016/04/State-of-the-Nation-report-web.pdf Accessed 12/22
16. NHS England. Future in mind: Promoting, protecting and improving our children and young people's mental health and wellbeing. *NHS England/Department of Health*, 2015. www.gov.uk/government/uploads/system/uploads/attachment_data/file/414024/Childrens_Mental_Health.pdf Accessed 12/22
17. Signorini G, Singh SP, Boricevic-Marsanic V, Dieleman G, Dodig-Ćurković K, Franic T, Gerritsen SE, Griffin J, Maras A, McNicholas F, O'Hara L, Purper-Ouakil D, Paul M, Santosh P, Schulze U, Street C, Tremmery S, Tuomainen H, Verhulst F, Warwick J, de Girolamo G; MILESTONE Consortium. Architecture and functioning of child and adolescent mental health services: A 28-country survey in Europe. *Lancet Psychiatry*. 2017 Sep;4(9):715–724. doi:10.1016/S2215-0366(17)30127-X. Epub 2017 Jun 6. Erratum in: *Lancet Psychiatry*. 2017 Dec;4(12):e29. Erratum in: *Lancet Psychiatry*. 2018 Feb 26. Erratum in: *Lancet Psychiatry*. 2019 Jul;6(7):e16. PMID: 28596067.
18. Blanz, B., and Schmidt, M. Practitioner review: Preconditions and outcome of inpatient treatment in child and adolescent psychiatry. *The Journal of Child Psychology and Psychiatry and Allied Disciplines*. 2000;41(6):703–712. doi:10.1111/1469-7610.00658

19. Rutter, M., Bishop, D., Pine, D., Scott, S., Stevenson, J. S., Taylor, E. A., and Thapar, A. *Rutter's child and adolescent psychiatry*. Hoboken: John Wiley & Sons, 2011.

20. Lewis, M. (Ed.). *Child and adolescent psychiatry: A comprehensive textbook*. Philadelphia: Lippincott Williams & Wilkins, 2002.

21. Semple, D., and Smyth, R. *Oxford handbook of psychiatry*. Oxford: Oxford University Press, 2013.

22. NICE. *Attention deficit hyperactivity disorder. Diagnosis and management of ADHD in children, young people and adults*. London: NICE, 2009a.

23. NICE. *Depression in children and young people. Identification and management in primary, community and secondary care*. London: NICE, 2005.

24. NICE and National Collaborating Centre for Mental Health. Self-harm. *The short term physical and psychological management and secondary prevention of self-harm in primary and secondary care*. London: NICE, 2004.

25. NICE, Bipolar disorder. *The management of bipolar disorder in adults, children and adolescents in primary and secondary care*. London: NICE, 2006.

26. The UK's Eating Disorder Charity – Beat, beateatingdisorders.org.uk Accessed 12/22

27. Medical Emergencies in Eating Disorders (MEED), www.rcpsych.ac.uk/improving-care/campaigning-for-better-mental-health-policy/college-reports/2022-college-reports/cr233. Accessed 12/22.

28. Volkmar, F. R., Lord, C., Bailey, A., et al. Autism and pervasive developmental disorders. *Journal of Child Psychology and Psychiatry*. 2004;45:135–171.

29. Young people's substance misuse treatment statistics 2020 to 2021: Report. *GOV. UK*, www.gov.uk Accessed 12/22.

30. Bruun, R. The natural history of Tourette's syndrome. In D. Cohen, R. Bruun, and J. Leckman (Eds.), *Tourettes syndrome and tic disorders*. New York: Wiley, 1988.

31. EAU. *Paediatric urology*. European Association of Urolog, 2019. www.uroweb.org

32. Encopresis in Children and Adolescents. Society of pediatric psychology, pedpsych.org Accessed 12/22.

7 Substance misuse and addictions

Arun Arujun Bhaskaran

Reasons for initiating substance use[1]:

- Genetics (positive family history, dopamine receptor gene polymorphisms).
- Personality (emotionally unstable personality disorder, antisocial personality disorder, novelty seeking and low impulse control traits).
- Social factors (low socioeconomic status, inner city/deprived areas, peer pressure).
- Mental illness.
- Childhood adversity and trauma, i.e., abuse.
- Cultural and religious attitudes.
- Ease of accessibility.
- Other factors, i.e., reduced educational attainment, unemployment/certain occupations, limited expectations.

Reasons for continuing use[2]:

1. Conditioning to certain cues and subsequent cravings.
2. Positive/negative (withdrawal effects) reinforcement.
3. Vicarious learning from peer pressure.

The reward pathway[3]

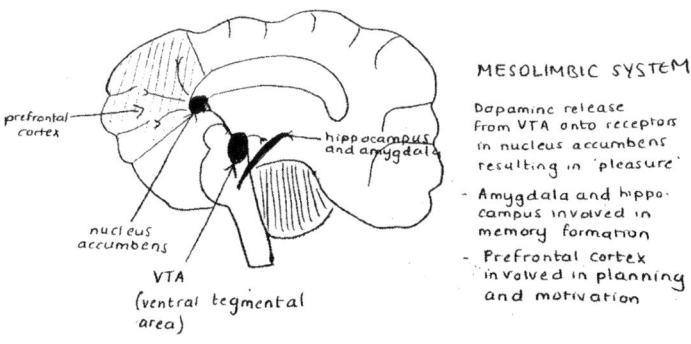

Figure 7.1 Reward pathways in the brain

DOI: 10.4324/9781003376163-7

Recognition of substance misuse

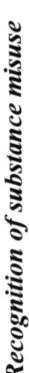

Structured assessment tools	Laboratory investigations	Bedside tests
CAGE (cutting down, angry, guilt, eye opener)	Liver function tests, gamma GT, clotting and full blood count in alcohol use	Urine drug screen Alcohol: 12-24 hrs Opiates: 1-3 days Cannabis: 1-3 days (episode), 30 days (dependent)
10-item AUDIT (alchol use identification test)		Ecstasy: 1-5 days Amphetamines: 2-4 days
SADQ (severity of alcohol dependence questionnaire)	Blood borne virus testing	Cocaine: 1-3 days Benzodiazepines: 3-7 days (episode), 30 days (dependent)

Physical examination (intoxication, withdrawal, stigmata of drug use)

Structured assessment tools

Laboratory investigations

Bedside tests (Breathalyser test for alcohol, UDS, hair analysis, oral fluid testing)

History taking

Recognition of substance use

Alcohol history

Type, frequency and quantity, age of onset, use over time, impact

Drug history

Types, frequency and quantity, age of onset, drug use history, impact

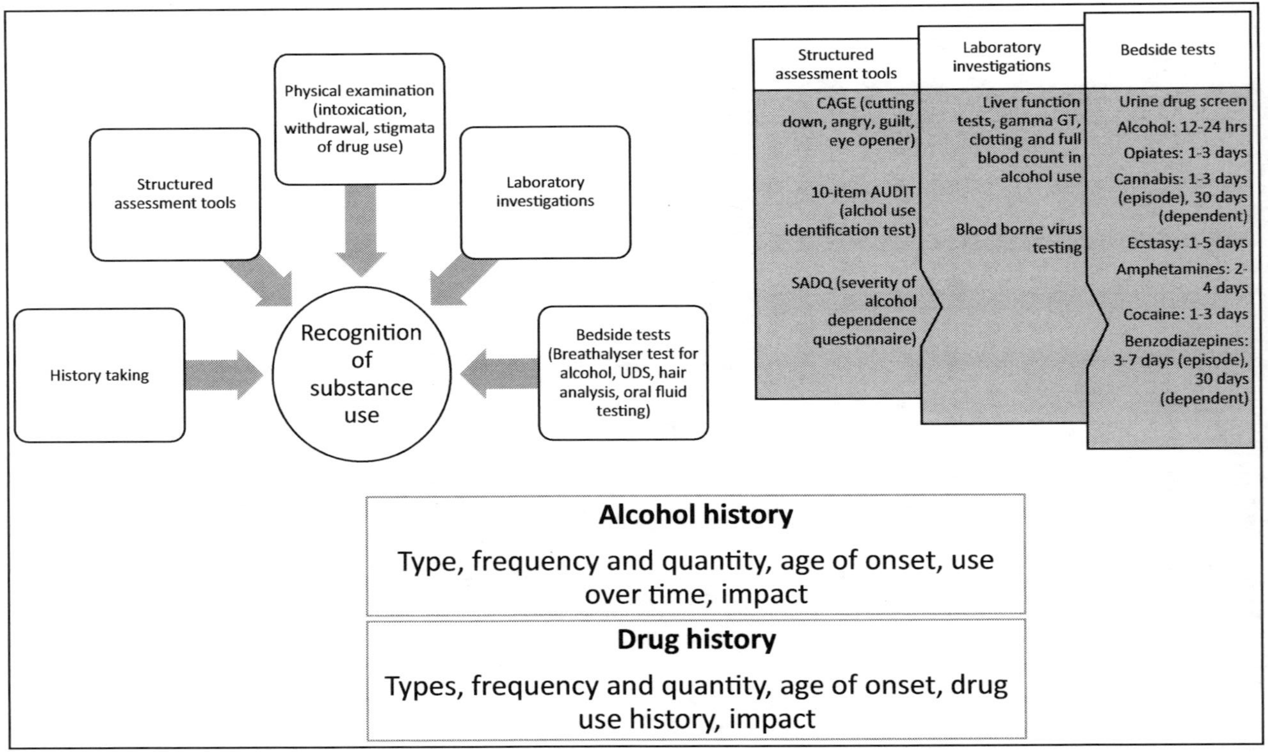

Figure 7.2 Recognition of substance misuse, points to elicit in a drug and alcohol history investigation, structured assessment tools and physical investigations

Patterns of substance use

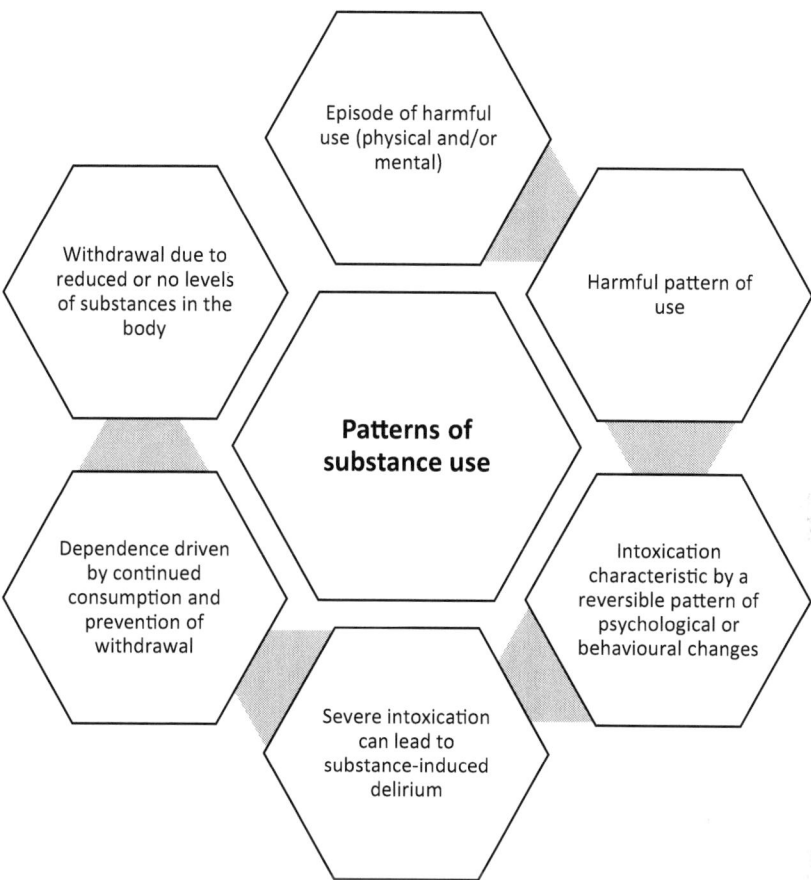

Figure 7.3 Patterns of substance misuse

Features of alcohol and substance dependence[4]:

1. Compulsions ('cravings').
2. Impaired control over use.
3. Tolerance (increasing doses required to achieve the same effect).
4. Continued use despite negative consequences.
5. Salience (prioritisation over other life aspects).
6. Narrowing of repertoire.
7. Rapid reinstatement following abstinence.

Related complications of alcohol and substance misuse[5]:

Table 7.1 Related complications of alcohol and substance misuse

Physical	• Malnutrition and dehydration. • Poor dentition. • Unsafe sexual practices. • Healthcare inequalities.
Psychological	• Greater rates of depression and anxiety. • Mental illness. • Higher prevalence of significant life events and past trauma. • Lack of trusting and confiding relationships and social isolation. • Greater risks through misadventure and impulsivity. • Suicide and self-harm, especially in intoxicated states.
Social	• Poor academic achievement leading to school drop-out and unemployment. • Peer exclusion, difficulties with relationships and social isolation. • Domestic abuse. • Financial difficulties. • Lack of stable accommodation and possible homelessness. • Difficulties accessing opportunities.
Public health	• Effects of unemployment and school drop-out. • Associated criminal practices. • Transmission of bloodborne viruses and sexually transmitted diseases (STDs). • Driving whilst under the influence of substances. • Accidents, including road traffic accidents. • Involvement in criminal activity. • Impact on NHS and healthcare services. • Children born to substance misusers and households using substances.

Interaction of drug and alcohol use with psychiatric illness:

- Idea of 'dual diagnosis'.
- Possible theories:

  - *Self-medication*
  - *Used to relieve stress and cope with adverse life events/trauma*
  - *Mental health sequelae of alcohol and substances*
  - *Overlapping vulnerabilities (positive family histories, genetic predisposition, psychosocial similarities including deprivation)*

Principles of substance misuse management:

- General considerations[6–8]:

  - *Service involvement*

- Shared care between general practitioners (GPs) and specialist services.
- Role of specialist drugs and alcohol services.

- Outpatient and inpatient management (including acute/psychiatric hospital, residential rehabilitation centres).

Psychoeducation:

- Provision for patients, family and friends.
- Counselling on physical health consequences including bloodborne viruses and STDs, dietary advice.
- Advice around driving and informing DVLA.

Treatment:

- Structured brief advice/extended brief interventions.
- Incorporation of motivational interviewing.
- Identification of goals with regular follow-up of progress.
- Community support networks and self-help groups (Alcoholics/Narcotics Anonymous).
- Signposting to charities.

Motivational interviewing[9–12]

Prochaska and DiClemente transtheoretical model ('Stages of Change'):

1. Pre-contemplation – individual not considering change.
2. Contemplation – individual is conflicted.
3. Preparation – individual collects information about change.
4. Action – individual works towards behavioural change.
5. Maintenance – individual continues behavioural change.
6. Relapse – individual returns to previous behaviours.

Processes of change move individuals between stages:

A. Experiential processes (early stages)

- Consciousness raising (increasing awareness of behaviours).
- Dramatic relief (increasing emotionality towards behaviours).
- Environmental re-evaluation (reassessing impact of behaviours on others).
- Self re-evaluation (reassessing impact of behaviour on self).
- Social liberation (belief that behaviour can change).

B. Behavioural processes (later stages)

- Stimulus control (minimising cues and triggers).
- Helping relationships (identifying appropriate social support).
- Counter-conditioning (identifying alternative behaviours).

- Reinforcement management (rewarding behavioural changes).
- Self-liberation (belief that maintenance of behaviour is possible).

Ambivalence can hinder behavioural change – conflict between short-term rewards and long-term consequences.

Miller and Rollnick's motivational interviewing (MI) is a type of counselling that helps reduce ambivalence and drive change. Meta-analyses show that MI is as effective or superior to other psychological/pharmacological interventions in substance misuse.

The 'spirit' of motivational interviewing (PACE):

- Partnership between therapist and client.
- Acceptance of client's thoughts, feelings and actions.
- Compassion towards client.
- Evocation of client's ideas.

Principles of motivational interviewing (DARES):

- Avoid arguments.
- Roll with the resistance.
- Empathise.
- Support self-efficacy.

Micro skills used in MI (OARS):

- Open-ended questions.
- Affirming.
- Reflecting.
- Summarising.

Ways to encourage 'change talk':

- Discuss disadvantages of the status quo.
- Consider advantages of change.
- Build optimism for change.
- Elicit intention to change.

Always consider whether a patient can 'commit' and is 'ready, willing and able' for change

Specific considerations:

Alcohol[13,14]

Alcohol use <15 units/day or AUDIT <20

- **Oral thiamine** and **dietary advice**.

- Individual psychological interventions (**CBT, behavioural, social network** and **environment-based**).
- **Behavioural couples therapy** for those with a regular and willing partner.

Alcohol consumption >15 units/day or AUDIT >20

1. Detoxification (medically-assisted withdrawal), ideally outpatient

   - Inpatient detoxification if **severe dependence, history of DT, comorbid mental or physical illness, learning disability/cognitive impairment** or **failed outpatient detoxes.**
   - **Fixed dose regimens in community settings.**
   - **Symptom-triggered** with monitoring via **Clinical Institute Withdrawal Assessment for Alcohol (CIWAA)** in inpatient settings.
   - **Chlordiazepoxide** or **diazepam** are drugs of choice.
     - *Lorazepam or oxazepam if liver impairment is present*

   - Prophylactic **parenteral thiamine** to prevent Wernicke encephalopathy (WE) and Korsakoff syndrome (KS).

     - *Note: glucose bolus in thiamine-deficient patients can precipitate WE*
   - Symptomatic relief (fluids for dehydration, antiemetics, haloperidol in delirium tremens).

2. Relapse prevention (therapies combined with pharmacological treatments)

   - **Acamprosate** (GABA analogue) to reduce **cravings.**
   - **Naltrexone** (opioid receptor blocker) to **inhibit reward pathway** with alcohol use.

     - *Avoid in acute liver failure and with patients taking opiates*

   - **Disulfiram** (ADH inhibitor) which causes **flush reaction** and negative reinforcement.

     - *Second line if other options not suitable*
     - ***Halitosis** can occur*
     - *Sudden-onset **jaundice** is a rare but important side effect*

Opiates[15–18]

1. Harm minimisation
- Psychoeducation
- **Needle exchanges** and accessibility to **blood-borne virus testing**.
- Pharmacological measures.

   - *Symptomatic relief for mild symptoms (loperamide, non-steroidal anti-inflammatory drugs [NSAIDs], prochlorperazine)*

- *Opiate substitution therapy (OST)*
  - *Requires **specialist initiation** and close monitoring*
  - ***Urine drug screen** and **Clinical Opiate Withdrawal Scale (COWS)** are helpful to ensure dependence*
  - ***Methadone** (long-acting μ receptor full agonist) or **buprenorphine** (long-acting μ receptor partial agonist)*
    - Methadone is associated with QTc prolongation (especially when taken with antipsychotics and cocaine) and **drug interactions** (especially CYP3A4 inducers/inhibitors)
    - Buprenorphine sublingual tablets can be injected and associated with greater **risks of diversion** (risk is lower with combined naloxone); methadone usually prescribed as 1 mg/ml oral solution
    - Buprenorphine can also induce a '**precipitated withdrawal**' with induction – out-competes full-agonist heroin and exerts a partial-agonist effect which patients perceive as withdrawal
    - OST can be prescribed at any time during pregnancy and is less harmful than continued illicit drug use – in third trimester, split dosing of methadone may be required due to faster metabolism
  - ***Slow-release oral morphine preparations (SROM)** and **dihydrocodeine** are used in exceptional circumstances*

2. Detoxification (outpatient/inpatient/residential)
   - Tolerance quickly diminishes following abstinence, so return to opioid use can trigger fatal overdoses.
   - **Naloxone** (opioid receptor antagonist) can reverse opioid overdose.

3. Relapse prevention
   - **Naltrexone** may have a role.
   - Psychological therapies.

Benzodiazepines[15]

Detoxification often involves switching to longer-acting drugs such as **diazepam**.

Substance addictions

Table 7.2 Specific substances and related clinical knowledge

	Epidemiology	Pharmacology	Route(s)	Effects	Intoxication	Withdrawal
Alcohol[19-21]	• In the UK, 24% of the population drinks over recommended amount and there are 602,391 dependent drinkers. • Binge drinking is a major problem in the UK (especially amongst younger population) and has led to changes in bars/pubs opening hours. • Worldwide, responsible for 5.3% of all deaths. • Societal factors, including social norms, economic development, availability and enforcement of policies (i.e., prohibition in certain Muslim countries). • Dependence peaks in middle age with a male preponderance (age discrepancy less amongst younger users). • Individual risk factors incl. family history, ethnicity, occupation, low socioeconomic status and psychiatric comorbidities.	• Rapidly absorbed from GI tract. • Water-soluble. • Peak levels reached in ~30 mins. • Metabolised in liver to acetaldehyde and then oxidised to acetate by alcohol dehydrogenase and microsomal ethanol-oxidising system (MEOS). • East Asians susceptible to flush reaction due to ALDH polymorphism.	• Oral.	*Physical* • Alcoholic fatty liver disease leading to cirrhosis and liver failure. • Chronic pancreatitis. • Gastritis, oesophageal varices and GI bleeding. • Dilated cardiomyopathy, arrhythmias. • Foetal alcohol syndrome. *Psychiatric* • Alcoholic hallucinosis, Othello syndrome. • Wernicke-encephalopathy with confusion, ataxia and ophthalmoplegia. • Korsakoff's syndrome – amnesia.	• Dysarthria. • Anxiolysis. • Impulsivity, disinhibition. • Respiratory depression. • Coma and death.	*3–12 hrs post last drink* • Tremors, nausea and vomiting, tachycardia, sweating. *12–18 hrs post last drink* • Grand mal seizures. *72–96 hrs post last drink* • Delirium tremens (DT).

(Continued)

Table 7.2 (Continued)

	Epidemiology	Pharmacology	Route(s)	Effects	Intoxication	Withdrawal
Opiates including heroin[22-24]	• Past trauma, dysfunctional communities and unemployment appear to be important factors. • Prescribing practices have led to increases in misuse. • Heroin use appears to be declining in younger populations (possibly due to public health warnings and witnessing long-term impact). • Increasing users receiving treatment including OST. • Past epidemics in the UK due to availability.	• Natural derivative of opium/synthetic substance that binds endogenous G-protein coupled μ and κ receptors which normally bind endorphins and encephalins. • Activation of receptors leads to hyperpolarisation, inhibition and reduced neurotransmitter release.	• Heroin (diamorphine) can be smoked ('chasing the dragon') or snorted. • With dependence, IV use develops. • Users inject subcutaneously (skin popping) or even intramuscularly when IV access becomes difficult.	IV use associated with: • Abscesses. • Deep vein thrombosis. • BBVs. • Sepsis. • Infective endocarditis.	• Euphoria, relaxation and analgesia. • Consider overdose in those with reduced Glasgow Coma Score, pinpoint pupils, respiratory depression and bradycardia. • Neonatal abstinence syndrome.	• 'Runs' – diarrhoea, vomiting, rhinorrhoea. • Yawning. • Piloerection. • Myalgia. • Hyperalgesia.
Cannabis[25-27]	• Most commonly abused illegal drug in the UK. • Rising patterns of use especially amongst younger populations. • Use often starts in school. • Increasing cannabis liberation worldwide (medicinal use of cannabis and legalisation). • Risk factors include alcohol and polydrug misusers and patients with mental illness (self-medicating).	• Metabolised by liver – 11-hydroxy-THC responsible for its effects. • Lipid soluble and accumulates in adipose tissue resulting in prolonged release and long half-life (up to a month). • Binds to endogenous cannabinoid receptors.	• Usually smoked (combined with tobacco to form a spliff) as a cigarette or a water pipe; can be consumed orally in food/drink but bioavailability lower due to first-pass hepatic metabolism.	Physical • Smoking can cause lung damage (cancers, chronic bronchitis) • Cerebrovascular damage • Mental effects • Psychosis (increased risks if younger age and heavier use) • Depression	• Anxiety and panic attacks. • Paranoia, derealisation, perpetual disturbances. • Euphoria. • Increase appetite ('munchies'). • Tachycardia. • Bloodshot eyes.	• Insomnia with vivid dreams. • Irritability. • Difficulties concentrating.

NMDA (ecstasy)[28,29]	• Commonly abused amongst younger populations; used at music concerts and festivals. • Reduced prevalence post-pandemic –related to reduced social contact.	• Has amphetamine and mescaline properties. • Metabolised by CYP2D6 – this displays genetic polymorphism and 'slower metabolisers' may be at risk of toxic effects. • Peaks around 1 hour after ingestion and effects last 4–6 hours. • Promotes the release of serotonin. • Also prevents the reuptake of dopamine and noradrenaline.	• Usually ingested orally (tablets/powder).	• Euphoria, increased alertness and feelings of increased mental abilities. • Dilated pupils. • Bruxism. • Diaphoresis. • Serotonin syndrome. • Severe hyperthermia and heat stroke. • Rhabdomyolysis and multi-organ failure. • Hyponatraemia and cerebral oedema (from drinking excessively to prevent heat stroke).	• Chronic exposure can result in neurotoxicity and associated: • Severe depression. • Memory and other cognitive impairment. • Paranoia.	• No specific withdrawal syndrome.
Gamma-hydroxybutyrate[30]	• Commonly abused amongst younger population especially party-goers. • Used by body builders as a supplement and also to facilitate arousal for sexual intercourse. • Increasingly used as a 'date-rape' drug due to its odourless and colourless properties.	• GBL is metabolised to form GHB which in turn is a precursor for GABA. • Fatty acids are highly lipophilic resulting in rapid onset of action. • Facilitates dopamine and glutamate release in a biphasic manner (results in both sedative and stimulant effects).	• Oral (liquid most commonly). • Sold as 'sushi soy fishies'.	• Euphoria, increased libido, disinhibition. • In higher doses can lead to high levels of vomiting, seizures, hypothermia and sedation (increased risks with concurrent alcohol use).	• Chronic use associated with depression, psychosis and cognitive impairment.	• Waxing and waning alcohol withdrawal-like syndrome with marked delirium and hallucinations.

(Continued)

Table 7.2 (Continued)

	Epidemiology	Pharmacology	Route(s)	Effects	Intoxication	Withdrawal
Amphetamines[31,32]	• Appears to have steadily declined in prevalence in the UK. • Often initiated to combat tiredness, improve attention or as a supplement for weight loss.	• Promotes release of noradrenaline, dopamine and serotonin. • Also inhibits reuptake transporters increasing levels in the synaptic cleft. • Commonly used are D-amphetamine, methylamphetamine (ice, crystal meth) and prescription-only appetite suppressants phentermine and diethylpropion. • Pemoline (brand name Cylert) was previously prescribed for ADHD but discontinued due to severe hepatotoxicity.	• Oral. • Snorted. • Methamphetamine can be smoked. • Injection possible and associated with higher risk of tolerance.	• Persistent dry mouth can lead to poor dental hygiene. • Severe weight loss. • 'Amphetamine psychosis' (hallucinations and paranoia). • Aggression and violence. • Anxiety, depression. • Reduced immunity and frequent infections.	• Sympathomimetic (dry mouth, tachycardia, hypertension, diaphoresis, dilated pupils). • Increased focus and alertness. • Anorexia. • Higher doses associated with irritability, aggression and paranoia. • Risk of cardiac arrhythmias and stroke (bleeds, embolism).	*24–48 hrs (crash phase)* • Increased urge to sleep, increased appetite *(withdrawal)* *1–2 weeks (withdrawal)* • Depression-like picture with mood swings, anhedonia, disturbed REM sleep with vivid dreams and anxiety *3–4 weeks (extinction)*

Cocaine[33,34]	• UK is the 'cocaine capital' of Europe. • Powder cocaine is the most commonly abused substance in the UK after cannabis (crack cocaine use may be underreported due to user lifestyle). • Increasing prevalence. • Used to be associated with wealth and certain professions – street costs have dropped sharply due to the deterioration of purity. • Manufactured in Bolivia, Colombia and Peru and trafficked throughout Central America.	• Binds and blocks DAT transporter releasing in reduced dopamine reuptake; also promotes dopamine release from the nucleus accumbens. • Rapid onset of action but short-lived duration results in compulsions and bingeing.	• Snorted. • Crack cocaine can be smoked. • Injection.	• 'Crack lung' (progressive fibrosis). • Necrosis and septal perforation from snorting. • 'Cocaine psychosis' (formication delusions 'cocaine bugs').	• When used with heroin can increase high ('snowballing'). • Stimulant effect. • Sympathomimetic. • Risk of heart attacks and strokes. • Agitation.	• Similar to amphetamines. • Marked cravings and drug seeking behaviours.
Hallucinogens[35,36]	• Use less common compared to other drugs. • Prevalence highest amongst young adults. • Certain hallucinogens are used in certain cultural practices and have a role in religious and spiritual rituals – condoned in certain governmental policies.	• Onset of action can be delayed but duration is prolonged with certain hallucinogens like LSD. • LSD binds serotonin receptors (5HT1, 5HT2, 5HT5 and 5HT7) and also facilitates dopamine release.	• LSD usually impregnated on 'tabs' and taken orally. • Magic mushrooms (psilocybin) can be consumed as food or drink. • Peyote (mescaline) and DMT can be made into tea (ayahuasca).	• Psychosis. • Flashbacks. • Hallucinogen persisting perception disorder (HPPD).	• 'Trips' ('bad trips') can be unpleasant). • Synaesthesia and changes in sense of time. • Dilated pupils but minimal other sympathomimetic effects. • Risks from chaotic behaviour due to altered reality.	• Limited research into dependence.

(Continued)

Table 7.2 (Continued)

	Epidemiology	Pharmacology	Route(s)	Effects	Intoxication	Withdrawal
Dissociative drugs[35]	• Limited research, but like hallucinogens, dissociative drugs play a part in religious, cultural and spiritual practices across the world, especially in parts of South America.	• PCP and ketamine are non-competitive NMDA receptor blockers. • Some effect on noradrenaline and endogenous opiate receptors. • Ketamine is degraded fully by first-pass metabolism if taken orally. • Shorter duration of action compared to hallucinogens.	• PCP (phencyclidine) can be ingested orally (capsules, liquid, white powder). • Ketamine powder can be snorted or injected and liquid can be ingested orally. • Salvia is endemic to parts of Central and South America and its leaves are chewed or dried and smoked.	• 'Ketamine bladder' is described with incontinence. • Speech difficulties and memory impairment have been described.	• Similar to hallucinogens but with marked sympathetic effects. Nystagmus, ataxia and delirium may occur. • Also 'out of body' and 'near death' experiences (described as entering the 'K-hole' with ketamine). • Risks from chaotic behaviour due to altered reality.	• Not described.

Benzodiazepines[37]	• Prescribing practices led to significant rates of misuse and dependence especially amongst females and older populations. • De-prescribing practices have led to increased deaths due to illegal sourcing. • Increased import and domestic production have also led to increased accessibility. • Significant rates amongst polysubstance users.	• Positive allosteric modulators on GABA-A receptors (ligand gated chloride channel). • Increase levels of GABA, which has a sedative effect on the brain. • Highly protein-bound and distributed throughout the body. • Complete bioavailability orally. • Lipid-soluble ATOM (alprazolam, triazolam, oxazepam, midazolam) drugs have the shortest onset times and half-lives and the greatest risk of misuse.	• Oral (tablets).	• Rebound insomnia and anxiety with prolonged use. • Panic attacks, agoraphobia and vivid nightmares have also been described.	• Sedation and induction of sleep. • Slurred speech. • Hypnotic and anxiolytic effects. • Mild memory impairment. • Euphoria in higher doses.	• Abdominal cramps and nausea. • Dizziness. • Headaches. • Tinnitus. • Blurred vision.
Barbiturates	• Less frequently abused since introduction of benzodiazepines.[38]	• Bind to different receptor sites on the GABA-A receptor.	• Oral or parenteral (especially IV).	• Mood swings. • Incoordination. • Poor concentration.	• Cerebellar-like picture CNS depression Respiratory depression can be fatal.	• Similar to alcohol withdrawal including seizures and delirium.

(Continued)

Table 7.2 (Continued)

	Epidemiology	Pharmacology	Route(s)	Effects	Intoxication	Withdrawal
Volatile inhalants[39]	• Predominantly used by adolescents with a mean age around 15 years. • Cheap and widely available. • Often misused after school and during school holidays. • Commonly due to peer pressure.	• Actions on the neuroglial membrane.	• Substances like adhesives, aerosols, cleaning solvents, fuel gases (butane, propane) and nitrous oxide are placed in a bag and fumes allowed to build before being 'huffed' or 'sniffed'.	• Cerebellar dysfunction. • Lead-containing inhalants can lead to cognitive deterioration. • Liver damage. • Peripheral neuropathies (from B12 deficiency) especially with nitrous oxide. • Perioral dermatitis. • Smell/stains on clothing.	• Euphoria. • Perceptual changes. • Laryngospasm, arrhythmias and cardiac arrest from vagal stimulation.	• Limited evidence available.

New psychoactive substances (NPS)[40]	• Previously known as 'legal highs' but now illegal to supply, sell or import.
	• Police now able to stop and search those suspected of these activities and can press charges (up to 7 years imprisonment)
	• Now under the control of the Misuse of Drugs Act 1971 and Psychoactive Substances Act 2016
	• Mimic the effect of illegal drugs
	  • Stimulants – i.e., BZP, mephedrone
	  • Hallucinogens – i.e., nitrous oxide
	  • Synthetic cannabinoids – i.e., Spice, Black Mamba
	  • Hallucinogens – i.e., 25i-NBOMe					

Non-substance addictions[41,42]

- **Gambling disorder:** pattern of online/offline gambling behaviour over 12 months resulting in impaired control, harm and continued use despite harm.
- **Gaming disorder:** pattern of online/offline gaming behaviour over 12 months resulting in impaired control, harm and continued use despite harm.
- **Other specified disorders due to addictive behaviours.**
- **Problematic internet use** and **online gaming.**
- **Compulsive shopping.**
- **Compulsive sexual activities.**
- **Excessive physical exercise.**
- **Binge eating.**

References

1. Altman J et al. The biological, social and clinical basis of drug addiction: commentary and debate. *Psychopharmacology*, 1996, 125, 285–345.
2. Wright P, Stern J, Phelan M. Core psychiatry, 3rd edition. London: Saunders Elsevier, 2012.
3. www.simplypsychology.org/brain-reward-system.html Accessed 04/22
4. Becker HC. Alcohol dependence, withdrawal, and relapse. *Alcohol Research & Health*, 2008, 31(4), 348–361.
5. GBD 2020 Alcohol Collaborators. Population-level risks of alcohol consumption by amount, geography, age, sex, and year: A systematic analysis for the Global Burden of Disease Study 2020. *Lancet*, 2022, 400(10347), 185–235.
6. Kaner EFS, Beyer FR, Muirhead C et al. *Effectiveness of brief alcohol interventions in primary care populations (Review)*. John Wiley & Sons, Ltd, 2018. www.cochranelibrary.com
7. NICE. Coexisting severe mental illness and substance misuse. *Quality Standard [QS188]. National Institute for Health and Care Excellence*, 2019. www.nice.org.
8. Department of Health. *UK Chief Medical Officers' low risk drinking guidelines*. London: Department of Health, 2016.
9. Rollnick S, Butler CC, Kinnersley P, Gregory J, Mash B. Motivational interviewing. *BMJ*, 2010, 340, c1900. doi:10.1136/bmj.c1900
10. Miller WR, Moyers TB. Motivational interviewing and the clinical science of Carl Rogers. *Journal of Consulting and Clinical Psychology*, 2017, 85(8), 757–766.
11. Miller WR, Rollnick S. *Motivational interviewing: Helping people to change* (3rd ed.). New York: Guilford Press, 2013.
12. Miller WR, Rollnick S. Ten things MI is not Miller, WR, Rollnick, S. (2009) Ten things that MI is not. *Behavioural and Cognitive Psychotherapy*, 2017, 37, 129–140.
13. NICE. *Alcohol use disorders: Diagnosis, assessment and management of harmful drinking and alcohol dependence. Quick reference guide*. London: National Institute for Health and Clinical Excellence, 2011a.
14. BNF. *British National Formulary*. London: National Institute for Health and Care Excellence (NICE), 2022.
15. Taylor DM, Barnes TRE, Young AH. *The Maudsley prescribing guidelines in psychiatry*. Hoboken: John Wiley and Sons Ltd, 2021.
16. NDSA. *National guidelines for medication-assisted treatment of opioid dependence*. Canberra: National Drug Strategy Australia, 2014.

17. NICE. *Drug misuse: Opioid detoxification*. London: National Institute for Health and Care Excellence, 2019a.
18. WHO, UNODC and UNAIDS. *WHO/UNODC/UNAIDS position paper. Substitution maintenance therapy in the management of opioid dependence and HIV/AIDS prevention*. Geneva: World Health Organization; United Nations Office on Drugs and Crime, 2006.
19. BMJ Best Practice. *Alcohol-use disorder*. London: BMJ Publishing Group, 2018.
20. ONS. *Alcohol-specific deaths in the UK: Registered in 2020*. London: Office for National Statistics, 2021.
21. www.who.int/news-room/fact-sheets/detail/alcohol Accessed 03/22
22. OHID. *Adult substance misuse treatment statistics 2020 to 2021: Report*. London: Office for Health Improvement and Disparities, 2021.
23. NHS Digital. *Statistics on drug misuse: England, 2018 (November update)*. London: NHS Digital, 2018.
24. BMJ. *Opioid use disorder*. London: BMJ Best Practice, 2019.
25. Office of the European Union. *European Monitoring Centre for Drugs and Drug Addiction, European drug report 2021: Trends and developments*. Luxembourg: Publications Office of the European Union, 2021
26. Connor JP, Stjepanović D, Le Foll B, Hoch E, Budney AJ, Hall WD. Cannabis use and cannabis use disorder. *Nature Reviews Disease Primers*, 2021, 7, 16.
27. Figueiredo PR, Tolomeo S, Steele JD, Baldacchino A. Neurocognitive consequences of chronic cannabis use: A systematic review and meta-analysis. *Neuroscience & Biobehavioral Reviews*, 2020, 108, 358–369.
28. Leung KS, Cottler LB. Ecstasy and other club drugs: A review of recent epidemiologic studies. *Current Opinion in Psychiatry*, 2008, 21(3), 234–241. doi: 10.1097/YCO.0b013e3282f9b1f1. PMID: 18382220.
29. https://hospitalhandbook.ucsf.edu/13-mdma-ecstasy-intoxication/13-mdma-ecstasy-intoxication Accessed 03/23
30. https://cpdonline.co.uk/knowledge-base/safeguarding/gamma-hydroxybutyric-acid/ Accessed 03/22
31. www.talktofrank.com/drug/speed Accessed 03/23
32. www.drugwise.org.uk/amphetamines/ Accessed 03/23
33. www.gov.uk/government/publications/united-kingdom-drug-situation-focal-point-annual-report/uk-drug-situation-2019-summary Accessed 03/23
34. https://nida.nih.gov/publications/drugfacts/cocaine Accessed 03/23
35. https://nida.nih.gov/research-topics/psychedelic-dissociative-drugs Accessed 03/23
36. Doyle MA, Ling S, Lui LMW, Fragnelli P, Teopiz KM, Ho R, Di Vincenzo JD, Rosenblat JD, Gillissie ES, Nogo D, Ceban F, Jawad MY, McIntyre RS. Hallucinogen persisting perceptual disorder: a scoping review covering frequency, risk factors, prevention, and treatment. *Expert Opinion on Drug Safety*, 2022, 21(6), 733–743. doi: 10.1080/14740338.2022.2063273.
37. Votaw VR, Geyer R, Rieselbach MM, McHugh RK. The epidemiology of benzodiazepine misuse: A systematic review. *Drug and Alcohol Dependence*, 2019, 200, 95–114. doi: 10.1016/j.drugalcdep.2019.02.033.
38. Skibiski J, Abdijadid S. Barbiturates. [Updated 2022 Dec 31]. In: *StatPearls [Internet]*. Treasure Island, FL: StatPearls Publishing, 2023. www.ncbi.nlm.nih.gov/books/NBK539731/
39. What are inhalants?. *National Institute on Drug Abuse (NIDA)*, nih.gov Accessed 03/23
40. www.gov.uk/government/publications/new-psychoactive-substances-nps-resource-pack Accessed 03/23
41. WHO. *International classification of diseases*, 11th Revision (ICD-11). Geneva: World Health Organization, 2022.
42. American Psychiatric Association. *Diagnostic and statistical manual of mental disorders* (5th ed.). Washington, DC: American Psychiatric Publishing, 2013.

8 Forensic psychiatry

Arun Arujun Bhaskaran

Crime is defined as an **intentional act** that causes **harm** or the **damage** or **destruction** of **property** and is **punishable** by **law**.[1]

Range of offences and specific crimes[2-4]

Table 8.1 Categories of criminal offences

Class	Sub-type	Definition
Homicide	**Murder**	Killing another person with the intention of killing or seriously harming them. Examples include: • Familicide: multiple-victim homicide (i.e., spouse and children). • Parricide: ones' parents (matricide – mother, patricide – father). • Siblicide: ones' siblings (fratricide – brother, sororicide – sister). • Honour killing: relative believed to have brought disgrace to family. • Murder-suicide: perpetrator's suicide within a week of committing homicide.
	Manslaughter	Killing another person without intending to actually kill them. Can be due to: • 'Reckless' behaviours. • Gross negligence. • Unlawful acts, i.e., speeding, drunk driving. • Serious mental illness. • Suicide pacts.

(Continued)

DOI: 10.4324/9781003376163-8

Table 8.1 (Continued)

Class	Sub-type	Definition
	Infanticide	• Neonaticide: intentional killing of a child up to 24 hours of age. • Infanticide: intentional killing of a child up to 12 months of age. • Filicide: occurs where a parent perpetrates infanticide. Reasons can include: • *Altruistic act to prevent suffering, i.e., terminally ill child* • *Psychosis or other serious mental illness* • *Unwanted child, i.e., unplanned pregnancy* • *Accident in the context of domestic abuse, etc.* • *Revenge*
Other violent crimes	**Common assault**	Deliberately or irresponsibly making someone believe that force is about to be used on them, where no unlawful contact is actually made, i.e., making verbal threats or displaying a weapon.
	Battery	Unlawful contact made to another which causes minor or no injury, i.e., spitting on someone, pushing someone.
	Actual bodily harm (ABH)	An assault leading to minor injury, i.e., punching someone and causing bruising or swelling.
	Grievous bodily harm (GBH)	An assault leading to serious injury, i.e., 'wounding' (injuries penetrating epidermis and dermis), fractures.
Sex offences	**Rape**	Intentional vaginal, anal or oral penetration with one's penis without another's consent.
	Assault by penetration	Intentional vaginal or anal penetration with a body part or 'anything else' for sexual purposes without another's consent.
	Harassment	Behaviour intended to cause another 'alarm or distress', i.e., sending unwanted correspondence, standing outside their place of residence; can be sexual in nature.
	Stalking	Persistently following someone (including through social media) invoking alarm or distress, disrupting functioning and impacting physical/mental health. Perpetrators include the: • 'Rejected', pursuing previous partners with whom they had been sexually intimate, or 'resentful', seeking revenge (some association with Cluster B personality disorders). • 'Intimacy seeking' (associated with high incidence of erotomania and delusional disorders). • 'Incompetent' with restricted social skills and understanding of relationships. • 'Predatory'.
	Sexual assault	Intentionally touching another person for sexual purposes without their consent.

Class	Sub-type	Definition
	Others	• Child sex offences – sexual communication with a child, causing a child to watch a sexual act, engaging in sexual activity in the presence of a child. • Indecent photographs of children, sexual exploitation of children. • Abuse of positions of trust. • Offences against a person with a mental disorder impeding choice, i.e., by care workers. • Prostitution, trafficking.
Criminal damage	**Fire setting**	Behaviours that can be accidental or intentional (could be criminal in nature). • Universal interest in fire in children, fire setting often due to curiosity in this age group. • Pathological fire setting due to psychological reasons can occur in personality disorders, psychosis, LD or acute intoxication from alcohol or drugs. • *Pyromania is a rare impulse control disorder described in the DSM-5 as 'deliberate and purposeful fire setting on >1 occasion' (with no instrumental gains or better explained by other diagnoses), 'tension or affective arousal before the act' and 'pleasure . . . when setting fires', as well as 'fascination with fire and . . . paraphernalia'*
	Arson	Criminal offence in which individuals willingly and maliciously set fire to or aid in setting fire to a structure, dwelling or property of another.
	Others	• Destroying or damaging property ('belonging to himself or another' 'without lawful excuse' and 'intending to . . . or being reckless'). • Threats to destroy or damage property • Possessing anything with intent to destroy or damage property

The relationship between mental illness and crime

There is an **ongoing debate** around the relationship between mental illness and crime. Studies highlight **links** between **different mental disorders** and **crime**, but links are **poorly understood** and estimates of risk vary between studies.

Other factors appear to be more strongly associated with criminality than mental illness alone,[5] including:

- **Male** gender.
- Age between **15 and 30 years**.
- **Past history** of criminality and violence.
- **Younger onset** of offending behaviour.
- **Socioeconomic deprivation**.

Overall, mental illness is considered a sole casual factor in **<10% of all crimes** committed. and the **vast majority** of individuals with mental illness will **never** engage in crime or violence.

There are concerns that attributing mental illness to criminal behaviour and violence can be **stigmatising, promoting negative attitudes and beliefs**.

Studies have highlighted how **mental health professionals, mass media** and **sensationalist reporting** can fuel these, particularly through language used, i.e., **'dangerous'** individuals.

Focus has shifted to the **vulnerabilities** of mentally unwell individuals and their roles as **victims** of crime, not perpetrators.[6–8]

- The **National Crime Survey** found that **40%** of patients with **severe mental illness** were victims of crime, compared to **14%** of the general population.
- Women with severe mental illness were **4 times** more likely to experience sexual violence and **10 times** more likely to experience any type of violence in the community.

Studies have also highlighted the impact of the criminal justice system on individual wellbeing (for example **prison psychosis**). The prevalence of post-traumatic stress disorder (**PTSD**) is also increased in mentally unwell offenders where criminal offences were **not premeditated** and patients were **disinhibited** at the time.[9]

Specific mental conditions and crime

Table 8.2 Links between different mental conditions and crime

Substance misuse[13–15]	• Strong associations with criminality shown in research.
	• **Drug-related, violent** (homicide, manslaughter) and **driving offences** appear to be most strongly linked.
	• *Acquisitive crime (burglary, shoplifting) reported in individuals with heroin and crack cocaine dependence*
	• Singleton et al. found **63% of male** and **39% of female prisoners** misused **alcohol; 50% of male** and **33% of female prisoners** misused **drugs.**[10]
	• Substance misuse appears to **elevate the risk of violence** in those with mental illness (particularly psychoses and personality disorders).
	• **Alcohol** and **benzodiazepine** are linked to **disinhibition** and subsequent **violent offences.**
	• *Touhig et al. found that alcohol use is implicated in 60–70% of homicides, and 44% of crime victims describe their perpetrators as intoxicated at the time*[11,12]
	• **Ongoing substance misuse** can also predict **reoffending risk.**
Epilepsy[16]	• Rarely responsible for offending behaviour – when it is, **partial complex seizures** appear to be most implicated.
	• **'Sane' automatisms** can be used as a defence during seizures or the post-ictal phase.

- **Episodic dyscontrol syndrome** and **intermittent explosive disorder** are associated with electroencephalogram (EEG) changes and angry outbursts followed by violence with amnesia.
  - *Usually seen in young males with congenital malformations or following traumatic brain injuries*

Bipolar affective disorder

- **Limited** evidence linking bipolar disorder, violence and crime.
- Some studies suggest a weak association between bipolar disorder and **violent offending**, citing **impulsivity** and **disinhibition** during manic/hypomanic episodes as having possible roles.[17]

Schizophrenia[18–20]

- Studies have identified a **moderately increased** risk of violent crimes in certain patients with schizophrenia.
  - *It is of note that existing studies focus predominantly on **high-risk samples**, and more research is needed regarding patients living with schizophrenia in the community*
- Risks appear greatest in those with a history of **violence/ offending behaviour**, **non-compliance** with treatment for their schizophrenia and **concurrent substance misuse**.
  - *Fazel et al. found substance misuse comorbidity increased risks **4-fold**[20]*
  - *A quarter of psychotic disorders in prisoners are substance associated*
- Reasons suggested for the increased risks include **cognitive impairment** and **affective deficits** impacting empathy and impulse control.
  - *The **threat/control override (TCO)** phenomenon described by Link et al. suggests that aggressive and violent behaviours in individuals with schizophrenia may arise from fears of being harmed or controlled*

Neurodevelopmental disorders[21]

- Individuals with intellectual disability (ID) and autism spectrum disorder (ASD) are **over-represented** in the justice system.
  - *ARC England estimated that people with **ASD** are **7 times** more likely to have contact with the police*
  - *15% of young persons in police custody at any time have **ASD** and 30% have suspected **ID***
  - *Estimated that 10% of **prisoners** have **ID** and even more have specific learning difficulties like dyslexia[22]*
- Most offenders with intellectual disability appear to have **mild or moderate severity**.
- Past studies have highlighted associations between **ID** and **arson** and **sexual offences** (particularly against young males) and between **ASD** and **violent crimes** and **criminal damage**.
- **Challenging** or unusual **behaviours, reduced appreciation of societal norms, restricted theory of mind**, impaired **social-emotional reciprocity and increased vulnerability** to suggestion and exploitation have been highlighted as reasons for offending behaviours in individuals with ASD and ID.

(Continued)

Table 8.2 (Continued)

	• Individuals with neurodevelopmental disorders can find the criminal justice system confusing and challenging and struggle to effectively communicate and express themselves. • *Offenders with neurodevelopmental disorders are* **struggle to achieve release from** *prison,* **serve more time** *and have* **higher reoffending rates**

Personality disorders[23]	• Studies highlight the association between personality disorder (PD) and criminality, particularly in regards to **antisocial, narcissistic** and **emotionally unstable** sub-types.
	• Questions have been raised around **social constructivism** and possible **over-diagnosis**, especially given that 'a **low threshold for discharge of aggression, including violence**' is an ICD-10 diagnostic criteria for antisocial personality disorder (ASPD).
	   • *Suggestion that* '**psychopathy**' *with traits of* **callousness, impulsiveness** *and* **egocentric interpersonal functioning**, *rather than PD, is a greater predictor of risk*
	• **High prevalence** of PD in prisons, up to **50% of female** and **64% of male prisoners**
	   • *ASPD is most prevalent in males, followed by paranoid PD*
	• Individuals with PD tend to commit crimes against **known victims** (including healthcare professionals) and offences include violence, sexual offences and arson.

Suicide[24,25]	• Significant prevalence of **major depression** in prison populations in the UK and worldwide. • **Completed suicide** account for up to **50%** of deaths in prison, with **prevalence rising**. • **Hanging** *is the most common method* • Suicide attempts typically occur in the first **6 months** of imprisonment and more prevalent in **younger individuals** with **life sentences** and **concurrent substance misuse**.

Special syndromes[26,27]

Table 8.3 Specific psychiatric syndromes

Morbid jealousy (Othello syndrome)	• Beliefs around partner's infidelity held with delusional intensity and conviction. • Can occur in personality disorders or psychoses. • Associations with confirmatory behaviours (stalking, harassment), domestic violence and, in extreme cases, homicide.
Erotomania (de Clerambault syndrome)	• Belief that someone is in love with the person, held with delusional conviction. • Can occur in psychoses. • Associations with stalking and harassment progressing to violence if rejected.

Munchausen syndrome	• Factitious disorder posed on self with feigning of signs and symptoms to receive medical care. • Separate from malingering, where there is often a secondary material gain, i.e., time off work, etc. • Links with childhood trauma, including serious physical illness as a child and personality disorders. • Munchausen by proxy is a factitious disorder posed on others (typically a child).

Mental disorders and offending in special groups[28-30]

Table 8.4 Offending in different groups of offenders

Young offenders	• Minimum age of criminal responsibility (**MARC**) in England and Wales is **10 years**.
	   • *No minimum in the majority of US states, and 18 years in parts of South America*
	• Under the MARC, individuals cannot be arrested or charged with a crime but can be subjected to curfews, supervision orders and local authority care.
	• Between the ages of 10–17, offenders can be arrested and taken to youth courts.
	   • *Usually detained in young offenders' institutes, secure training centres or detention centres rather than 'prisons'*
	• Conduct disorder appears to be over-represented.
	• Estimated 50–70% of youths in the juvenile justice system meet criteria for a mental illness.
	• Increasing emphasis on youth prevention programmes and diversion of youths out of the justice system.

Female offenders	• Females in contact with the criminal justice system more often have **mental health difficulties, concurrent substance misuse** and are **victims of abuse**. • Females are prosecuted for **less severe offences – TV licence evasion** and **shoplifting** were the most common offences in recent statistics. Females tend to steal fewer items and items of lower value than male counterparts. • Females represent a smaller proportion of the **prison population** and on average serve **shorter sentences**. • A higher proportion of female prisoners **self-harm** in prison. • Females, on average, have **higher reoffence rates**.
Offenders from ethnic minority groups	• Latest UK figures suggest ethnic minorities are **over-represented** at most stages in the criminal justice process compared to Caucasians. • *The greatest disparities appear regarding **stop-and-searches, custodial remands** and **prison populations*** • **Black individuals** appear to be the most over-represented. • **Greater proportions** of prisoners <18 years are from ethnic minorities.

(Continued)

Table 8.4 (Continued)

	• Ethnic groups on average have **longer sentences** than their Caucasian counterparts. • This appears to mirror **restrictive mental healthcare practices** in ethnic minorities (more **detentions under the Mental Health Act** and higher rates of **seclusion** and **physical restraint**).
Deafness and physical disability	• May impact **accessibility** (physical environment, communication needs) at any stage in the criminal justice process. • May impact **fitness to plea**. • **Deafness** and **chronic ill health** may be associated with increased **mental health difficulties** and associated **mortality/ morbidity**.

Psychiatry and the criminal justice system

The role of the psychiatrist is the assessment of mentally disordered offenders at any point in their journey through the justice system.[27,31]

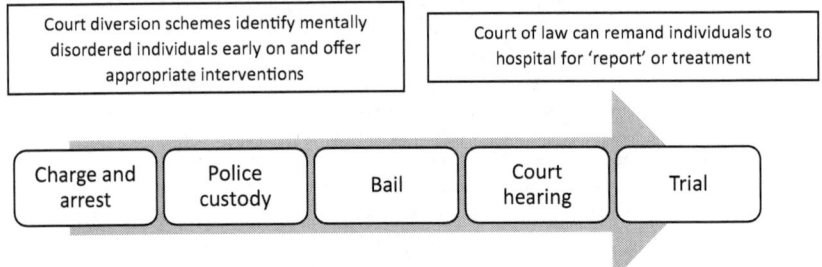

Figure 8.1 Journey through the criminal justice system

Criminal responsibility (accountability) = mens rea (guilty mind) + actus reus (voluntary act)

McNaughton's (M'Naghten) legal test for a defence of 'insanity'[32]*:*

> Every man is to be presumed to be sane, and . . . that to establish a defence on the ground of insanity, it must be clearly proved that, at the time of the committing of the act, the party accused was laboring under such a **defect of reason**, from **disease of mind**, and **not to know the nature and quality of the act** he was doing; or if he did know it, that he did **not know he was doing what was wrong**.

Individuals can be acquitted of charges or convicted for lesser offences if deemed 'not guilty by reason of insanity'.

Psychiatric defences[33]

A. *Fitness to plead*
   To stand a full trial, a defendant should fulfil the Pritchard criteria and:

- Understand the charges made against them.
- Decide whether to plead guilty or not guilty.
- Follow court proceedings.
- Instruct counsel.
- Provide evidence in their defence.
- Challenge a juror.

If found unfit to plead, a **trial of facts** can take place instead.

B. *Mutism and deafness*

C. *Diminished responsibility*
   In murder cases, individuals cannot be fully acquitted of the charges, but can be convicted of manslaughter (England, Wales) or culpable homicide (Scotland) instead.

D. *Amnesia*

- **Dissociative** or **organic** in nature.
- **Alcohol-** or **drug-induced amnesia** not considered due to motivation to escape liability through self-inducing.

E. *Automatisms*

- Acts that occur when individual is **unconscious** of **grossly impaired** consciousness and unaware that an act is occurring.
- Can be '**sane**' (due to extraneous factors, i.e., severe hypoglycaemia) or '**insane**' (due to endogenous factors, i.e., epilepsy, sleepwalking)

Disposals following conviction[33]

1. Full acquittal and **absolute discharge.**
2. **Conditional discharge** and **probation*.**
3. **Prison sentence**.**
4. **Hospital care***.**
5. **Supervision order** for treatment and support.
6. **Guardianship order** for care and protection.

   National Offender Management Service **(NOMS) links prison and probation services.*

**Individuals can be *transferred to hospital* at any point during their sentence if there are any mental health concerns.*

***Courts of law can impose *restriction orders* which prevent hospitals from authorising *leave* or *discharging* certain offenders without Ministry of Justice permission.*

Psychiatrists are expected to develop skills in writing court reports related to criminal cases and providing oral evidence in courts as professional and expert witnesses.

Practicing psychiatry in a secure setting

Role of security in a therapeutic setting[34]

Security aims to **protect** from **harm, uncertainty** and **anxiety**. Levels of security should be **proportional** to the risks and regularly reviewed.

Security in therapeutic settings centres on:

- **Overt risks** – i.e., absconding, violence and aggression.
- **Covert risks** – i.e., accessing sensitive information and contraband.

Levels of secure care settings:

- **High** – for individuals posing serious and immediate risks to others.
- **Medium** – for those posing serious but less immediate risks to others and risks of absconding.
- **Low** – for those posing less serious risks to others.
- Psychiatric intensive care units (**PICUs**) for shorter-term care.

Aspects of security:

- **Physical** – i.e., locked doors, high perimeter fences.
- **Procedural** – i.e., nursing observations, searches.
- **Relational** – i.e., training, communication between colleagues and patients.

Components of a forensic service and managing offenders in different settings

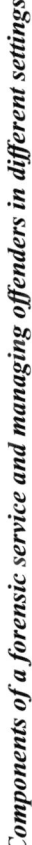

Psychiatric intensive care units (PICUs) for treatment of those posing acute risks to others in other inpatient settings

Low secure units for those who 'pose a significant danger to themselves and others'

Medium secure (regional secure) units for those who present a 'serious danger to the public'

Forensic outreach services providing consultation and liaison to general community mental and inpatient teams and prison in-reach

High secure hospitals like Broadmoor, Rampton and Ashworth for individuals with a 'grave and imminent danger'

Forensic services

Specialist community forensic teams (adult/CAMHS) with MDTs consisting of forensic psychiatrists, psychologists and nurses

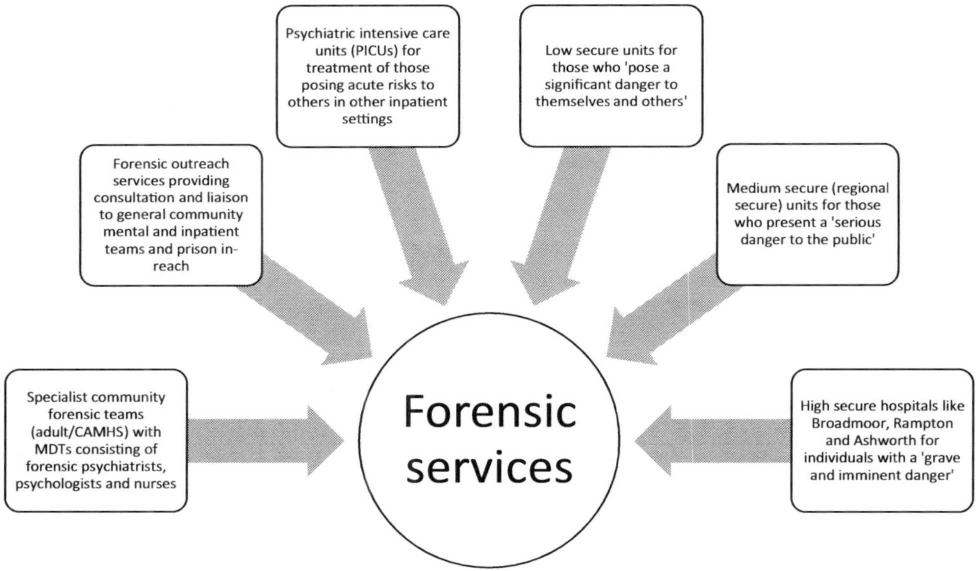

- Police and court liaison and diversion services, prison in-reach services and youth offending teams and charities link up the criminal justice system and specialist forensic services.
- Multi-Agency Public Protection Arrangements (MAPPA) link up professional agencies and ensure the successful management of high risk offenders particularly in cases of violent and sexual crimes.

Figure 8.2 Components of a forensic service and managing offenders in different settings.

Risk management planning in forensic psychiatric practice[35,36]

- **Risk is** defined as the 'likelihood of harm (physical or psychological) occurring'.
- **Risk elimination** is unachievable, so focus should be on **risk reduction**.

    - *This concept has driven incentives such as **paracetamol pack size limitation***

Examples of risks in psychiatric practice:

Risks to self	Risks to others
• Self-harm.	• Verbal aggression.
• Completed/suicide attempts.	• Physical aggression.
• Purging.	• Physical violence.
• Self-neglect.	• Property damage.
• Disengagement from services.	• Safeguarding towards adults and children.
• Non-compliance with treatment.	• Criminal offences.
• Disinhibition.	• Driving offence.
• Reputation.	• Disinhibition.
• Development and ability to thrive.	
• Social isolation.	
• Exploitation.	
• Physical health complications.	

Figure 8.3 Examples of clinical risk

Risk assessment aims to estimate risk of an untoward event occurring and forms an integral part of psychiatric practice that is particularly pertinent in forensic settings.

Aspects of a comprehensive risk assessment:

- Consideration of **static** (fixed and historical) and **dynamic** (fluctuating) risk factors.
- **History.**
- **Mental state examination.**
- **Intent.**
- **Planning.**
- **Risk formulation** covering the following:

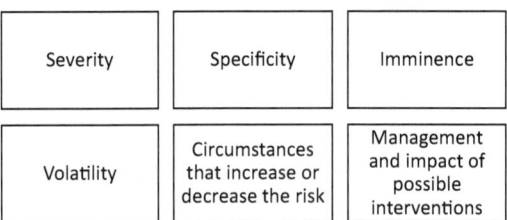

Figure 8.4 Risk formulation

Barriers to effective risk assessment[37]

1. Not lending sufficient weight to views of **carers** and the **general public**.
2. Undue emphasis on **civil liberties** of individuals and not correctly implementing the **Mental Health Act**.
3. Taking a **cross-sectional** rather than longitudinal perspective on risks.
4. Not appropriately **sharing information**.

Types of risk assessment[38]

Unstructured – based entirely on the clinician and usually shaped by their personal views, experience and instinct.
+ Flexible, individualised
– Low inter-rater reliability, low predictive value, low legal utility
Actuarial – algorithms are used to quantitatively determine risk.
+ Better inter-rater reliability and predictive value, recognised by policy-makers
– Poor generalisability, undue emphasis on static risk factors

Examples: Static-99 (sexual recidivism in adult male sex offenders), Level of Service Inventory (general recidivism in older adolescent and adult offenders) and Violence Risk Appraisal Guide-Revised (violence in offenders with mental illness).

Structured professional judgements aim to combine both actuarial and unstructured approaches.

Examples: Historical, Clinical and Risk-20 (violence), Sexual Violence Risk-20

Human rights legislation as it affects patients and psychiatric practice[39,40]

- The **European Convention on Human Rights** (ECHR) was established to protect the rights of people in the **Council of Europe**.
- The **Human Rights Act 1998** incorporates the rights established at the ECHR into British Law.

  - *Came into effect in **October 2000** and protects everyone in the UK*

- The Act organises human rights into **'articles'**:

Article 2: Right to life
Article 3: Freedom from torture and inhuman or degrading treatment
Article 4: Freedom from slavery and forced labour

> **Article 5:** Right to liberty and security
> **Article 6:** Right to a fair trial
> **Article 7:** No punishment without law
> **Article 8:** Respect for one's private and family life, home and correspondence
> **Article 9:** Freedom of thought, belief and religion
> **Article 10:** Freedom of expression
> **Article 11:** Freedom of assembly and association
> **Article 12:** Right to marry and start a family
> **Article 14:** Protection from discrimination in respect of these rights and freedoms

- **Public bodies**, including the NHS and the criminal justice system, must comply with the Act.
- Particularly pertinent articles relating to forensic practice include **Articles 5, 6** and **7**.

References

1. What is a crime? *Victim Support*, https://www.victimsupport.org.uk/crime-info/what-crime/#:~:text=-%20Victim%20Support%20What%20is%20a%20crime%3F%20A,a%20crime%20at%20some%20point%20in%20their%20lives Accessed 03/2023
2. Types of crime *Victim Support*, https://www.victimsupport.org.uk/crime-info/types-crime/ Accessed 03/2023
3. Common offences. *Sentencing*, sentencingcouncil.org.uk Accessed 03/2023
4. Crime type definitions. *Metropolitan Police*, https://www.met.police.uk/sd/stats-and-data/met/crime-type-definitions/ Accessed 03/2023
5. Tanner-Smith EE, Wilson SJ, and Lipsey MW. (2012) Risk factors and crime. In FT Cullen and P Wilcox (eds), *The Oxford Handbook of Criminological Theory*. Oxford: Oxford Academic.
6. Khalifeh H, Johnson SC, Howard LM, et al. (2015) Violent and non-violent crime against adults with severe mental illness. *British Journal of Psychiatry*, 1–8. Doi: 10.1192/bjp.bp.114.147843
7. Brennan IR, Moore SC, Shepherd JP. (2010) Risk factors for violent victimisation and injury from six years of the british crime survey. *International Review of Victimology* 17(2), 209–229
8. Office of National Statistics, www.ons.gov.uk/ Accessed 03/2023
9. Hanson R. et al. (2010) The impact of crime victimization on quality of life. *Journal of Traumatic Stress* 23(2), 189–197.
10. Singleton N, Meltzer H, Gatward, R. et al (1998) *Psychiatric Morbidity Among Prisoners in England and Wales*. London: HMSO.
11. Håkansson A, Jesionowska V. (2018) Associations between substance use and type of crime in prisoners with substance use problems – A focus on violence and fatal violence. *Substance Abuse and Rehabilitation* 9, 1–9. Doi: 10.2147/SAR.S143251.
12. Touhig DA. (1998) British All-Party Committee view on alcohol and violence. *Alcohol and Alcoholism* 33, 88–91.

13. Poole R, Brabbins, C. (1997) Substance misuse and psychosis. *British Journal of Hospital Medicine*, 58, 447–450.

14. Johns A. (1998) Substance misuse and offending. *Current Opinion in Psychiatry*, 11, 669–673.

15. Thomson LDG. (1999) Substance abuse and criminality. *Current Opinion in Psychiatry*, 12, 653–657.

16. Halle C, Tzani-Pepelasi C, Pylarinou N-R, Fumagalli A. (2020) The link between mental health, crime and violence. *New Ideas in Psychology*, 58, 100779. Doi: 10.1016/j.newideapsych.2020.100779.

17. Bipolar disorder and violent crime. *NICS Well*, https://www.nicswell.co.uk/health-news/bipolar-disorder-and-violent-crime Accessed 03/2023

18. Tsimploulis G, Niveau G, Eytan A, Giannakopoulos P, Sentissi O. (2018) Schizophrenia and criminal responsibility: A systematic review. *The Journal of Nervous and Mental Disease*, 206(5), 370–377. doi: 10.1097/NMD.0000000000000805.

19. Wallace C., et al. (2004) Criminal offending in schizophrenia over a 25-year period marked by deinstitutionalization and increasing prevalence of comorbid substance use disorders. *American Journal of Psychiatry*, 161, 716–727

20. Fazel S, Grann M. (2006) The population impact of severe mental illness on violent crime. *American Journal of Psychiatry*, 163, 1397–1403

21. http://hebw.cf.ac.uk/learningdisabilities/chapter6.htm Accessed 03/2023

22. Home – ARC England Accessed 03/2023

23. Davison S, Janca A. (2012) Personality disorder and criminal behaviour: What is the nature of the relationship? *Current Opinion in Psychiatry*, 25(1), 39–45. doi: 10.1097/YCO.0b013e32834d18f0.

24. Birmingham, L. (2003) Mental health of prisoners. *Advances in Psychiatric Treatment*, 9, 191–201

25. Fazel S, Danesh J. (2002) Serious mental disorder in 23 000 prisoners: A systematic review of 62 surveys. *The Lancet*, 359, 545–550.

26. Taylor A. (2000) *Faulk's Basic Forensic Psychiatry*, 3rd edn. Edited by J Stone, KO Shea, S Roberts. London: Blackwell Publishing

27. How a criminal case works, cps.gov.uk Accessed 03/2023

28. Eastman N, Adshead G, Fox S. (2012) *Forensic Psychiatry*. Oxford: Oxford University Press

29. www.gov.uk/age-of-criminal-responsibility Accessed 04/2023

30. www.gov.uk/government/statistics/women-and-the-criminal-justice-system-2021/women-and-the-criminal-justice-system-2021 Accessed 04/2023

31. www.gov.uk/government/statistics/ethnicity-and-the-criminal-justice-system-statistics-2020/ethnicity-and-the-criminal-justice-system-2020 Accessed 04/2023

32. Preparing for exams. *Royal College of Psychiatrists*, rcpsych.ac.uk Accessed 03/01/2023.

33. http://forensicpsychiatryexperts.co.uk/the-mcnaughton rules#:~:text=The%20McNaughton%20rules%20refer%20to%20the%20legal%20test,he%20incorrectly%20believed%20to%20be%20the%20Prime%20Minister Accessed 04/2023

34. Gunn J, Taylor PJ. (2013) *Forensic Psychiatry Clinical, Legal and Ethical Issues*, 2nd edn. London: Taylor and Francis.

35. www.nursingtimes.net/archive/delivering-security-focused-healthcare-22-03-2007/ Accessed 04/2023

36. Natarajan M, Srinivas J, Briscoe G, Forsyth S. (2012) Community forensic psychiatry and the forensic mental health liaison model. *Advances in Psychiatric Treatment*, 18(6), 408–415. doi:10.1192/apt.bp.109.006940

37. www.rcpsych.ac.uk/members/supporting-your-professional-development/ assessing-and-managing-risk-of-patients-causing-harm/assessing-risk   Accessed 04/2023.
38. Lipsedge M. (1995) Clinical risk management in psychiatry. In C. Vincent (ed), *Clinical Risk Management* (pp. 276–293). London: BMJ Publishing.
39. Kapur N. (2000) Evaluating risks. *Advances in Psychiatric Treatment*, 6(6), 399–406. doi:10.1192/apt.6.6.399
40. www.equalityhumanrights.com/en/human-rights/human-rights-act Accessed 04/2023

9   Disorders of intellectual development

Arun Arujun Bhaskaran

Definition[1]:

Group of conditions arising in the developmental period characterised by:

*   Significantly **limited intellectual functioning** across various cognitive domains AND
*   Significantly **limited adaptive behaviour** and difficulties in performance of:

    *   *Conceptual skills involving application of knowledge, i.e., reading and writing*
    *   *Social skills and communicating and interacting with others*
    *   *Practical skills to ensure independence including self-care, managing finances and maintaining safety AND*

*   May be associated with comorbid **physical, mental, neurodevelopmental** and **behavioural problems** or conditions.

Synonyms and previously used terminology:

*   *Disorders of intellectual development (ICD-11)*
*   *Learning disability (MRCPsych syllabus)*
*   *Learning difficulty (often used in education to refer to specific problems with learning)*
*   *Intellectual disability (DSM-5)*
*   *Developmental disability*
*   *Intellectual developmental disorder*
*   *Mental retardation (ICD-10)*
*   *Mental handicap*

DOI: 10.4324/9781003376163-9

Classification[2]

ICD-11 states that intellectual developmental disorders should be assessed using '**appropriately normed, individually administered standardised tests**'.

- **Mild** – intellectual functioning and adaptive behaviour 2–3 standard deviations below the mean (0.1–2.3th percentile).
- **Moderate** – intellectual functioning and adaptive behaviour 3–4 standard deviations below the mean (0.003–0.1th percentile).
- **Severe** – intellectual functioning and adaptive behaviour 4 or more standard deviations below the mean (<0.003rd percentile). Individuals may be able to speak a few words but have poor motor ability.
- **Profound** – intellectual functioning and adaptive behaviour 4 or more standard deviations below the mean (<0.003rd percentile). Individuals often have complex health requirements and most are non-verbal.

  - *Standardised intelligence tests cannot reliably/validly distinguish between severe and profound and clinical judgement is required*

Intelligence quotient (IQ) tests used in clinical practice[3]:

- **Stanford-Binet test** (original IQ test).
- **Wechsler scales** (WAIS-R for adults, WISC for children).
- **Raven's progressive matrices** account for cultural biases.

In terms of IQ:

- Mild: 50–69
- Moderate: 35–49
- Severe: 20–34
- Profound: <20

Social history of learning disability[15]:

- **Pre-17th century**
  - As early as Ancient Greece, affected individuals were considered to have a *'deleterious influence on developing societies and therefore needed to be eradicated'*.

- **17th century**
  - Under the **Elizabethan Poor Act**, these individuals were believed to be a threat to society and were locked away in 'poor houses'.

- **18–19th centuries**
  - The Industrial Revolution brought along with it the need for skilled labour and individuals with ID were not considered *'profitable members of society'*.
  - The **Poor Law Amendment Act** responded by placing them in 'workhouses'.

- **Early 19th century**
  - Individuals were termed 'feeble-minded' and believed to be responsible for crime and societal ills.
  - Growing ideology that 'feeble-mindedness' was hereditary and state control through **eugenics** was necessary.

- **1913**
  - The **Mental Deficiency Act** legalised the detention of 'idiots', 'imbeciles' and 'feeble-minded persons'.
  - Many individuals were institutionalised in **long-stay hospitals**.

- **20th century**
  - The **European Convention on Human Rights (1950), 'Better Services for the Mental Handicapped' White Paper (1971)** and the **Jay Report (1979)** highlighted the devastating impact of institutionalisation and stressed the importance of caring for individuals in the community.
  - **Normalisation** highlighted that individuals with intellectual disability have a right to the most 'culturally normative' lives possible, and this can be achieved through **social role valorisation** (inclusion and creating opportunities).

Epidemiology[4,5]

Prevalence and incidence of learning disability in the general population:

- **1.5 million people** live with a learning disability in the UK.
- **2.16%** of UK **adults** have a learning disability.
- **2.5%** of UK **children** have a learning disability.
- Most of those with a learning disability fall into the **mild** category (**profound** is the least common).
- Incidence hard to establish due to mild learning disability being unnoticed until later in life.

Prevalence and incidence of superadded impairments:

- Estimated prevalence of **mental health difficulties** ranges from **15–52%** depending on diagnostic criteria used.

Mental and behavioural comorbidities

- Schizophrenia.
- Mood and anxiety disorders.
- Autism spectrum disorder (ASD) and attention deficit hyperactivity disorder (ADHD).
- Dementia.
- Conduct disorder.
- Behaviour that challenges.

- Studies also show that individuals with a learning disability are at greater risk of **physical health conditions** and have poorer outcomes due to **inequalities in healthcare**. There is also a risk of **diagnostic overshadowing** and attributing physical health symptoms to symptoms of a learning disability.

  - *Life expectancies of women and men with learning disability are* **18 and 14 years shorter**, *respectively, than those of the general population.*

Physical health comorbidities

- Sensory impairments, particularly visual and hearing.
- Dental disease.
- Weight concerns and malnutrition.
- Epilepsy and other neurological problems.
- Musculoskeletal and mobility issues.

- Biological factors, higher rates of negative life events, health inequalities, reduced coping skills and internalised stigma may be contributing factors.
- **Increasing severity** appears to increase the risk of superadded impairments.

Aetiology[6]

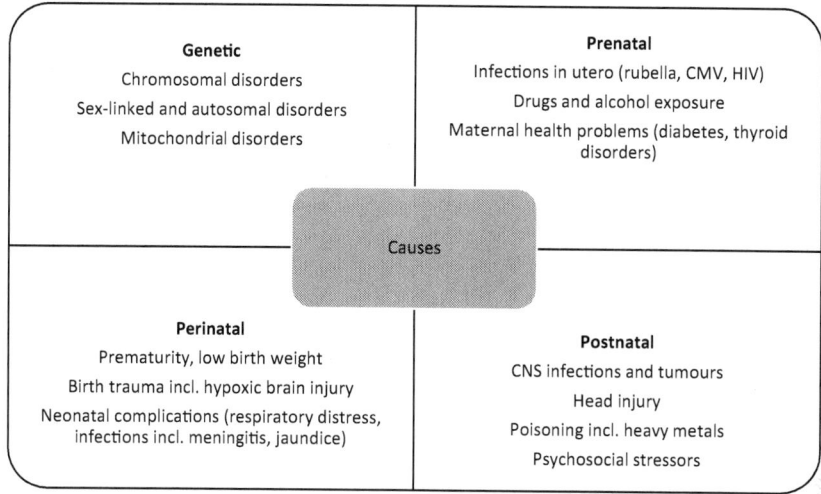

Figure 9.1 Risk factors for learning disability

Common genetic conditions associated with learning disability[7–10]

Table 9.1 Common genetic conditions associated with intellectual disability

Syndrome	What you need to know
Down	• Most common chromosomal disorder, ~1 in 1000 births.
	• Caused by presence of all or part of an extra chromosome 21 (majority due to nondisjunction at meiosis but can be due to a Robertsonian translocation, mosaicism or duplication).
	• *Increased risk with increasing maternal age*
	Clinical features include:
	• *Dysmorphic features – hypotonia, epicanthic folds, oblique palpebral fissures, open mouth with protruding tongue, low-set ears, depressed nasal bridge and occiput, single palmar crease and sandal toe deformity*
	• *Physical health conditions – cardiac defects, duodenal atrea, imperforate anus, tracheo-oesophageal fistula, Hirschsprung disease, hypospadias, cryptochorchism, orthopaedic disorders, cataracts, obesity, asthma, obstructive sleep apnoea and leukaemia*
	• *Neurodevelopmental and psychiatric problems – learning disability of varying severity (average IQ 50), ASD, ADHD, challenging behaviour and Alzheimer's disease*
	• Usually picked up during prenatal screening (serum beta-hCG and nuchal translucency scanning) and confirmed with chorionic villus sampling or amniocentesis.

(Continued)

Table 9.1 (Continued)

Syndrome	What you need to know
	• Management requires an individual multidisciplinary treatment (MDT) approach to screen, diagnose and treat complications. • Prognosis improved with better healthcare and follow-up – congenital heart disease is the biggest cause of mortality. Early-onset Alzheimer's dementia common cause of morbidity.
Edward	• Trisomy 18. • Characterised by intrauterine growth retardation, microcephaly, rocker-bottom feet, clenched fists with over-riding fingers, absent thumbs and cardiac/renal abnormalities. • Prognosis poor, with majority dying *in utero* or by first year of life.
Patau	• Trisomy 13. • Characterised by microphthalmia, cleft lip/palate, cardiac and brain/spinal cord abnormalities. • Prognosis poor, with majority dying by first year of life.

DiGeorge (velocardiofacial)	• 22q11 deletion.
	• Characterised by:
	  • *Mild dysmorphic features – cleft lip/palate, wide nasal bridge, short philtrum and velopharyngeal insufficiency*
	  • *Physical health conditions – congenital heart disease, hypoparathyroidism/hypocalcaemia and T-cell immunodeficiency*
	  • *Neurodevelopmental and psychiatric problems – mild to moderate learning disability and increased risk of schizophrenia*

Williams-Beuren (Williams)	• 7q11.23 deletion (elastin and LIM kinase-1 genes implicated).
	• Characterised by:
	  • *Dysmorphic features – wide mouth with a pronounced bottom lip and widely spaced teeth, upturned nose and high cheeks*
	  • *Physical health conditions – supravalvular aortic stenosis common and hypercalcaemia common*
	  • *Neurodevelopmental and psychiatric problems – strong verbal skills with excessive talking and uninhibited behaviour with mild to moderate learning disability*

Smith-Magenis	• 17p11.2 deletion. • Characterised by severe insomnia, ADHD, mild to moderate LD, self-injurious and aggressive behaviours.
Wolf-Hirschhorn	• 4p deletion. • Characterised by 'Greek helmet' dysmorphic features, epilepsy and learning disability of varying severity.

Cri-du-chat	• 5p15.2 deletion
	• Characterised by:
	  • *Dysmorphic features tend to become less prominent with age (round face with hypertelorism and prominent epicanthal folds)*
	  • *Characteristic high-pitched cry as an infant*
	  • *Neurodevelopmental and psychiatric problems – severe to profound intellectual disability, ADHD, self-injurious and aggressive behaviours*

Syndrome	What you need to know
Rubinstein-Taybi	• 16p13.3 deletion. • Moderate-severe LD, OCD, ADHD symptoms and expressive language difficulties common.
Neurofibromatosis type 1 (Von Recklinghausen)	• Autosomal dominant mutation in NF1 gene encoding neurofibromin. • Lisch nodules in the iris, café au lait spots and neurofibromas are characteristic. • Increased risk of ADHD and learning disability of varying severity.
Tuberous sclerosis	• Autosomal dominant mutation in TSC1/TSC2 genes encoding hamartin and tuberin. • Angiofibromas, ungula fibromas, shagreen patches, ash-leaf macule, infantile spasms and non-cancerous hamartomas in eye, kidney and heart occur. • ASD with or without ADHD can occur along with intellectual disability of varying severity.
PKU	• Autosomal recessive disorder resulting in build-up of phenylalanine. • Hypopigmentation of skin and characteristic musty odour. • Reversible cause of severe LD – diet and medication.

Fragile X	• Mutations in FMR1 gene.
	• Affects both males and females, but females tend to have milder symptomatology.
	• Characterised by:
	  • *Dysmorphic features including long and narrow face, large ears, flat feet and macro-orchidism*
	  • *Physical health conditions including seizures*
	  • *Neurodevelopmental and psychiatric problems: developmental delay especially in speech and language, learning disability of varying severity, ASD and ADHD*
	• Normal IQ.
	• Short stature, broad chest with widely spaced nipples.

Turner	• 45, X. • Normal IQ. • Short stature, broad chest with widely spaced nipples and webbed neck.
Klinefelter	• 47, XXY. • Specific learning difficulties, i.e., dyslexia. • Tall stature.
Usher	• Associated with deafness and psychosis.
Prader-Willi	• Associated with deletions on the paternal chr15. • Associated with lack of appetite satiety leading to obesity, hypogonadism and IQ <70. • Psychosis is also seen.
Angelman	• Associated with deletions on the maternal chr15. • Associated with happy disposition, hand flapping and clapping and severe/profound LD.

(*Continued*)

Table 9.1 (Continued)

Syndrome	What you need to know

Lesch-Nyhan	• X-linked recessive disorder leading to HGPRT deficiency and uric acid accumulation.
	• Presentation:
	  • *Physical health – abnormal motor movements, seizures, renal failure*
	  • *Mental health – uncontrollable self-injury and aggression*

Hunter	• X-linked recessive disorder leading to iduronate sulfatase deficiency and glycosaminoglycan accumulation. • Neurodegenerative disorder and can cause hearing loss, cardiac abnormalities, loss of speech, ADHD symptoms and LD.
Congenital hypothyroidism	• Reversible cause of LD, presents with symptoms of hypothyroidism.
Corneila de Lange	• Mutations of NIPBL gene on chr5. • Distinguishing facies include hypertrichosis, long philtrum and small hands and feet. • Associated with self-injurious and aggressive behaviours.

Foetal alcohol spectrum disorder	• Greatest risk with regular heavy drinking and binge drinking during pregnancy.
	• Characterised by:
	  • *Dysmorphic features that do not remit with age – short palpebral fissures, flat smooth philtrum and thin upper lip*
	  • *Growth deficiency – microcephaly and short stature*
	  • *Mild LD, speech and language difficulties, ADHD, visuospatial and memory impairment*

Presentation, assessment and diagnosis[11–13]

General considerations in diagnosing mental illness in individuals with learning disability:

- Diagnostic criteria based on studies that don't include this demographic.
- Available assessments not robust.

   - *Psychiatric Assessment Schedule for Adults with Developmental Disabilities (**PAS-ADD**) and the **mini PAS-ADD** can be helpful*

- Impairments might make it difficult for individuals to express what is going on for them.
- Presentation can be very different and more subtle, i.e., change in behaviour.

Challenging behaviour – daily behaviours that cause more than minor injury to self or others or the destruction of property, causes more than a few minutes disruption and requires intervention – occurs in 7% of LD population, M>F.

- When signs and symptoms present, they tend to be attributed to learning disability – **diagnostic overshadowing**.

Presentation of specific mental health conditions in individuals with learning disability:

- **Psychosis** – talking to self or having imaginary friends might be developmentally appropriate for some individuals with LD. Individuals might experience struggles expressing thoughts and appear tangential/distractible/thought-disordered, paranoia due to stigma and discrimination or preoccupation with others.
- **Bipolar disorder** – does not typically present as mania (hyperactivity, challenging behaviours, i.e., wandering, aggression).
- **Depression** – impairments in abstract thought might make affective symptoms difficult to express and suicidality is rare, may present as regression/self-injurious behaviours/anhedonia.
- **Dementia** – early detection may be difficult due to baseline impairments, atypical symptoms common and include transient psychosis, late-onset epilepsy and nocturnal confusion.

Points to consider when communicating with individuals with learning disability[14]:

- Consider **environmental factors** such as noise/light levels in the room, where you and the individual are positioned, etc.
- Use clear and **straightforward language** – avoid jargon or long words.
- Use **concrete** examples.
- Use different **methods** and **formats** (written, signing, visual imagery, practical demonstrations).
- Check for **understanding**.
- Go at the **individual's pace** and follow their lead.
- Involve **carers** and **advocates**.

Treatment

Specialist services[11–13]:

- Introduction of specialist LD teams to aid normalisation, reduce health inequalities and improve access.
- MDT approach.
- Support general teams to enhance care for those with mild to moderate LD and care for those with more severe conditions.

Psychological treatments:

- **Behavioural approaches** are most commonly used.

  - *Functional analyses consider antecedents, behaviours and consequences (ABC) and can be helpful understanding challenging behaviours*

- **CBT** and **psychotherapy** also used.
- Modified approaches due to communication impairments and limited abstract thought.
- **Systemic approaches** involving family and carers is important considering the biopsychosocial impact of having a child with a disability on the family (guilt, inferiority, tension and conflict between partners and siblings, health anxieties, carer fatigue).

Drug treatments

- Trends of over-usage and polypharmacy.

  - *Review medications regularly and stop inappropriate prescriptions*

- Prescribing in more severe LD should be undertaken and supervised by specialist teams.
- Physical comorbidities should be considered carefully.

  - *For example, medications may lower seizure thresholds or interact with anticonvulsants in those with comorbid epilepsy*

- Increased sensitivities to adverse effects (particularly antipsychotics and anticholinergics), so a 'start low and go slow' approach is used with dose titrations.

Specific treatments:

Table 9.2 Specific medications used for comorbid conditions in those with LD

Methylphenidate	• Comorbid ADHD.
Naltrexone	• Severe and refractory self-injurious behaviours.
	• Studies inconsistent.
Valproate	• Strongest evidence for mood stabilisation.
Lithium	• Self-injurious behaviours.
	• Rapid-cycling bipolar affective disorder.
SSRIs	• Obsessional thoughts, severe anxiety (esp. in ASD).
	• Risk of hypomania.
Low dose antipsychotics	• Risperidone best evidence base.
	• Psychotic illness, challenging behaviours.
	• Increased risk of metabolic syndrome long-term.

References

1. https://cks.nice.org.uk/topics/learning-disabilities/background-information/definition/ Accessed 11/2022
2. https://icd.who.int/browse11/l-m/en#/http://id.who.int/icd/entity/605267007 Accessed 11/2022
3. Drozdick L., & Puig, J. (2019). Intellectual assessment. In M. Sellbom & J. Suhr (Eds.), *The Cambridge Handbook of Clinical Assessment and Diagnosis* (Cambridge Handbooks in Psychology, pp. 135–159). Cambridge: Cambridge University Press. doi:10.1017/9781108235433.012
4. www.mencap.org.uk/learning-disability-explained/research-and-statistics/how-common-learning-disability#:~:text=Approximately%202.16%25%20of%20adults%20in%20the%20UK%20are,951%2C000%20adults%20with%20a%20learning%20disability%20in%20England. Accessed 11/2022
5. Smiley E. (2005). Epidemiology of mental health problems in adults with LD. *Advances in Psychiatric Treatment*, 214–223
6. Bhate S., & Wilkinson S. (2006). Aetiology of learning disability. *Psychiatry*, 5(9), 298–301, https://doi.org/10.1053/j.mppsy.2006.08.001.
7. Wright P., Stern J., & Phelan M. (2012). *Core Psychiatry*, 3rd edition. London: Saunders Elsevier.
8. Gardiner M., Eisen S., & Murphy C. (2009). *Training in Paediatrics – The Essential Curriculum*. London: OST.
9. BeaPttie M., & Champion M. (2012). *Essential Revision Notes in Paediatrics for the MRCPCH*, 3rd edition. Knutsford, UK: Pastest.
10. Liassauer T., & Clayden G. (2012). *Illustrated Textbook of Paediatrics*, 4th edition. London: Mosby Elsevier.
11. Emerson (1995). *Cited in Emerson, E (2001, 2nd edition): Challenging Behaviour: Analysis and Intervention in People with Learning Disabilities*. Cambridge: Cambridge University Press.
12. Gelder, M., Gath, D., & Mayou, R. (1989). *Oxford Textbook of Psychiatry* (2nd ed., pp. 681–725). Oxford: Oxford University Press.
13. Rogers, A. E. (2004). *Companion to Psychiatric Studies. Sociology & Psychiatry* (6th ed.). Amsterdam, Netherlands: Elsevier B.V.
14. www.mencap.org.uk/learning-disability-explained/communicating-people-learning-disability Accessed 11/2022
15. https://langdondownmuseum.org.uk/the-history-of-learning-disability/social-history-of-learning-disability/ Accessed 11/2022

10 Critical review

Arun Arujun Bhaskaran

Evidence-based medicine is the 'conscientious, explicit and judicious use of current best evidence in making decisions about care of individual patients', and trainees should be **actively assessing scientific literature** rather than passively absorbing facts from 'experts'.[1]

Processes involved in evidence-based medicine:

1. Identify a **clinical question**.
2. Find **available evidence** and **review** it.
3. **Apply** evidence.
4. **Assess** the **clinical impact**.

Clinical questions may be related to:

Table 10.1 Categories of clinical question

Aetiology	Does drinking red wine increase the risk of Alzheimer's dementia?
Diagnosis	Is the Connor's questionnaire a useful tool in diagnosing ADHD?
Therapy	Is venlafaxine superior to mirtazapine in the treatment of refractory depression?
Economic	Which service is more cost-effective in rural Cumbria – domiciliary or outpatient clinics?
Harm	Can prophylactic procyclidine prevent the onset of extrapyramidal side effects with haloperidol use?
Prognosis	What vulnerability factors increase the risk of relapse in psychotic depression?
Meaning	What are service users' experiences with virtual psychology appointments?

Translation of clinical uncertainty into an answerable question[2,3]

2 types of clinical question:

- **Background** – *general* knowledge about a condition, test or treatment, i.e., what are the clinical features of catatonic schizophrenia?

DOI: 10.4324/9781003376163-10

- **Foreground** – asking for *specific* information to aid clinical decision making.

Use the **PECOT formula** to devise foreground questions:

Table 10.2 Components of the PECOT formula

P	Patient	Who is your target population?
E	Exposure	What is the treatment you are considering?
C	Comparison	What are you comparing the exposure against?
O	Outcome	What is the impact?
T	Time	How long will it take to achieve this?

Good clinical questions enable you to select the best **evidence-based practice tools** to search for evidence and select **filters** in databases to refine searches.
Systematic retrieval of the best available evidence[4]:

1. Ask a **clinical question**.
2. **Critically review** existing literature and make **hypotheses**.
3. Design a **study** and **recruit test subjects**.
4. Carry out study and **collect data**.
5. **Analyse** the data.

Different sources of evidence:

Types of study:

- **Observational studies** do not make changes to the subjects' environments.

  - *Descriptive studies describe patterns and trends between subjects*
  - *Analytical studies offer explanations for these patterns and trends*

- **Experimental studies** make changes to subjects' environments and assess the impact of these changes.

Table 10.3 Types of study

Study type	Description	Clinical question
Case report	Describes an isolated case.	
Case series	Describes a small group of individuals.	
Case control	Compares healthy and affected persons and looks retrospectively to consider aetiological factors.	Therapy, harm, aetiology
Cross-sectional	Looks at individuals at a single point in time and considers any similarities and differences.	Aetiology, diagnosis

(*Continued*)

Table 10.3 (Continued)

Study type	Description	Clinical question
Cohort	Follows a group of individuals over time to investigate how they are impacted by a disease.	Prognosis
Ecological	Follows larger populations rather than individuals or smaller groups.	
Quasi-experimental	Considers the relationship between different variables without random sampling methods.	Therapy, harm, aetiology
Randomised controlled trial	Makes use of random sampling methods to determine relationships between variables – can be in experimental or pragmatic settings.	Therapy, harm, aetiology
Systematic review	Gathers results of all available studies in a particular area to produce a comprehensive summary.	
Meta-analysis	Uses statistical methods to summarise the results of multiple studies.	
Economic studies	Compare the costs and impacts of different healthcare interventions.	Economic
Qualitative research	Produces non-numerical data.	Meaning

'The hierarchy of evidence'[5]:

Systematic reviews and **meta-analyses**, followed by **randomised controlled trials**, are considered rigorous sources of evidence, whereas **expert opinions, anecdotal evidence** and **background information** are not.

GRADE, SIGN and the **Oxford Centre for EBM** provide different grading systems to assess how 'good' a study is.

Electronic databases[6]:

Table 10.4 Different types of electronic database

Cinahl (Cumulated Index to Nursing and Allied Health Literature)	Nursing and allied health sciences.
Cochrane Library[7]	Systematic reviews and meta-analyses.
EMBASE (Excerpta Medica database)	Pharmacology.
PsycInfo	Psychology research papers.

| Pubmed (Medline) | Main database for published medical research. |
| Sigle (System for Information on grey literature) | 'Grey literature' (government documents, annual reports, white papers, etc. |

Strategies for efficient evidence retrieval from databases[7]:

- Define clinical question using **PECOT**.
- Identify appropriate **electronic database** and **study types**.
- Conduct an **explosive search** initially then **filter**.
- Make use of:
    - Boolean operators (AND, OR, NOT).
    - Truncation/stemming (i.e. nurs* for nurse, nurses and nursing).
    - Wildcard (i.e. wom?n for woman or women).
    - Quotation marks around phrases i.e. 'COVID pandemic'.
    - Parentheses/nested parentheses i.e. ((mouse or rat) AND trap) or mousetrap).

Figure 10.1 Strategies for effective evidence retrieval

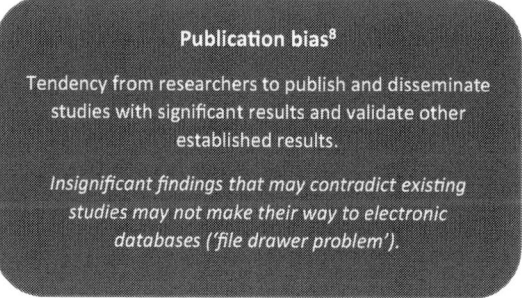

Publication bias[8]

Tendency from researchers to publish and disseminate studies with significant results and validate other established results.

Insignificant findings that may contradict existing studies may not make their way to electronic databases ('file drawer problem').

Figure 10.2 Publication bias[8]

Critical appraisal of the evidence

Basic epidemiology[9]

Epidemiology is defined as **the study of how frequently diseases** occur in **different populations** and **why** (*aetiology*).

- The **total population** encompasses every individual in an area.
- Researchers will be interested in a **target population**, i.e., those with a particular health condition or a certain type of medication.

- Only the **accessible population** will be available to researchers (those who may be willing to take part and meet the inclusion criteria).
- **Samples** are derived from the **accessible population**.

Sampling[10]

- A **census** involves studying every single individual within a population. This can be expensive and time-consuming.
- **Sampling** involves studying a portion of the population.

Probability sampling methods (every member of the population has an equal chance of being chosen):

1. *Simple random* – using random number generators/other methods to pick individuals at random.
2. *Stratified random* – dividing a population into groups and randomly selecting individuals from each group.
3. *Block random* – dividing a population into 'blocks', randomly selecting some blocks and recruiting some individuals from each randomly.
4. *Cluster random* – dividing population into 'clusters', randomly selecting some and recruiting all individuals in selected clusters.
5. *Systematic random* – ordering individuals and selecting every n^{th} member.

Non-probability sampling methods (every member of the population does not have an equal chance of being chosen):

1. *Convenience* – selecting easily accessible individuals in the population.
2. *Voluntary response* – picking those who volunteer for the study.
3. *Snowball* – recruiting a few initial individuals and asking them to recruit more participants.
4. *Purposive* – selecting individuals from the population who is felt to be the most useful for the study.

Concepts used to evaluate the quality of studies[11]:

Table 10.5 Definitions of accuracy, precision, validity and reliability

Accuracy	The degree of closeness of study measurements to actual measurements.
Precision	The degree of closeness between study measurements.
Validity	The degree to which a study investigates what it intended to investigate internally (amongst sample subjects and within study conditions) and externally (to other samples/populations and 'real life conditions). Can be: • *Face validity – surface level* • *Construct validity – ideas/theories* • *Content validity – all aspects of the construct(s)* • *Criterion validity – correlation to existing study outcomes (concurrent); ability to predict related outcomes (predictive)*

Reliability   The degree to which results can be consistently replicated.
- *Inter-rater reliability – uniformity of results amongst different researchers*
- *Test-retest reliability – uniformity of results over time*

Some errors within studies can occur via chance (**random errors**) and can be difficult to control for, whereas some can be due to the study design or quality and can be amended (**systematic errors/bias**).[12]

Table 10.6 Types of systematic errors

Type of systematic error	Sub-type	Description
Reporting – occurs when reviewing existing literature and hypothesising	Outcome reporting	Studies selectively reporting some findings and not others.
	Language	Studies being published only in certain languages.
	Duplicate	Repeated publication of certain findings.
	Time lag	Delayed publication of certain studies.
	Dissemination	Findings never being published.
	Location	Certain studies being hard to find (no electronic copies, unavailable on electronic databases).
Selection – occurs when recruiting and allocating subjects	Response	Characteristics of volunteer subjects differing from those of the population.
	Membership	Subjects belonging to a certain group (like in snowball samples).
	Historical	Subjects being recruited over time.
	Diagnostic purity	Subjects with comorbidities being excluded from studies.
	Berkson	Subjects being recruited from inpatient settings.
	Nyman	Delays between subject recruitment and onset of disease.
Performance		Usually due to instruments or tools used during the study.
Observation – occurs during data gathering	Interviewer	Un-blinded researchers altering their findings.
Can be limited by blinding subjects	Recall	Subjects selectively remember certain details and not others.
(single) or subjects and researchers (double)	Response	Subjects responding in a way they believe researchers want them to.
	Hawthorne	Alteration in subjects' behaviour due to the awareness of being observed.
Analysing data – occurs when reviewing data and drawing conclusions	Attrition	Many subjects drop out of the study.

***Basic biostatistics*[13]**

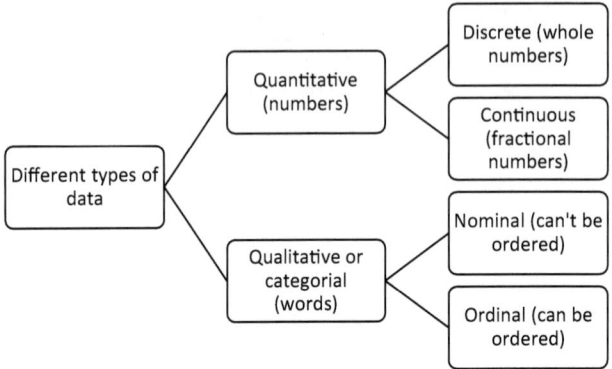

Figure 10.3 Types of data

Data summary measures:

Table 10.7 Data summary measures

Lower quartile	Value 1/4 of the way through the data set
Median	Middle value
Upper quartile	Value 3/4 of the way through data set
Mode	Most common value

The following are the spelling test scores out of 20 for a group of students in a Year 4 class:

3, 4, 4, 4, 5, 5, 6, 7, 8, 8, 9, 10, 11, 11, 12, 12, 13, 13, 16, 17, 18, 19, 19, 20, 20, 20

Mean ($\bar{x}$) – sum of data values/number of data values = 294/26 = 11.3
Median – 11
Upper quartile – 17
Lower quartile – 6
Mode – 4 and 20

Measures of data spread:

Table 10.8 Measures of data spread

Range	Highest value – lowest value.
Interquartile range	Upper quartile – lower quartile.
Variance	Sum of (data value – mean) squared/ number of data values – 1.
Standard deviation	√variance.

Consider the earlier example:

Table 10.9 Worked example of data spread

x	$\bar{x}$	$x - \bar{x}$	$(x - \bar{x})^2$
3	11.3	$3-11.13 = -8.3$	68.89
4	11.3	$4-11.3 = -7.3$	53.29
4	11.3	$4-11.3 = -7.3$	53.29
4	11.3	$4-11.3 = -7.3$	53.29
5	11.3	$5-11.3 = -6.3$	36.69
5	11.3	$5-11.3 = -6.3$	36.69
6	11.3	$6-11.3 = -5.3$	28.09
7	11.3	$7-11.3 = -4.3$	18.49
8	11.3	$8-11.3 = -3.3$	10.89
8	11.3	$8-11.3 = -3.3$	10.89
9	11.3	$9-11.3 = -2.3$	5.29
10	11.3	$10-11.3 = -1.3$	1.69
11	11.3	$11-11.3 = -0.3$	0.09
11	11.3	$11-11.3 = -0.3$	0.09
12	11.3	$12-11.3 = 0.7$	0.49
12	11.3	$12-11.3 = 0.7$	0.49
13	11.3	$13-11.3 = 1.7$	2.89
13	11.3	$13-11.3 = 1.7$	2.89
16	11.3	$16-11.3 = 4.7$	22.09
17	11.3	$17-11.3 = 5.7$	32.49
18	11.3	$18-11.3 = 6.7$	44.89
19	11.3	$19-11.3 = 7.7$	59.29
19	11.3	$19-11.3 = 7.7$	59.29
20	11.3	$20-11.3 = 8.7$	75.69
20	11.3	$20-11.3 = 8.7$	75.69
20	11.3	$20-11.3 = 8.7$	75.69
Total $(x - \bar{x})^2$			829.54

Range – 20–3 = 17
Interquartile range – 17–6 = 11
Variance – 829.54/(26–1) = 829.54/25 = 33.18
Standard deviation – $\sqrt{33.18}$ = 5.76

Tabular and graphical presentations:

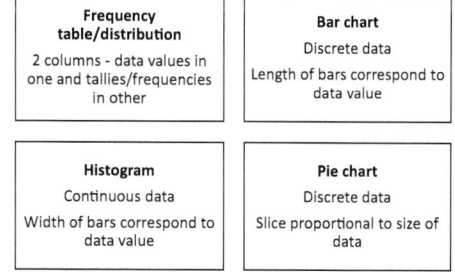

Figure 10.4 Types of tabular and graphical presentations

Box plot:

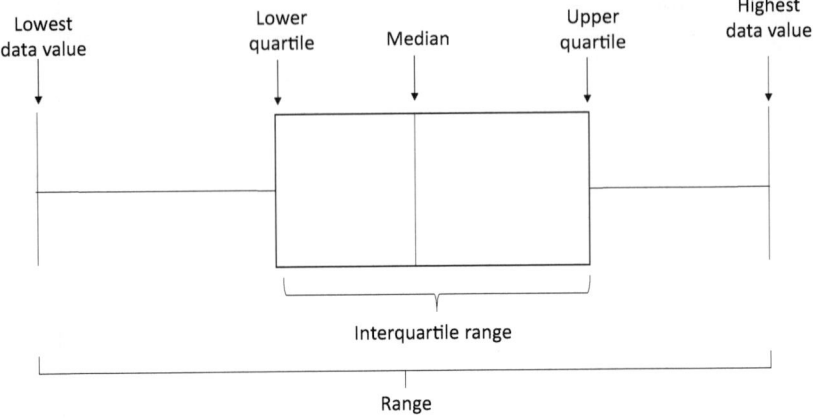

Figure 10.5 Components of a box and whisker plot

Diagnostic tests[14]

- **Gold standard** tests provide a benchmark that is regarded as definitive, i.e., *oral glucose tolerance tests for diabetes.*
- These tests can be **impractical, unpleasant** or **expensive**, so there is a need for other diagnostic screening tests.

Table 10.10 Definitions of true positives, false positives, false negatives, true negatives, sensitivity, specificity, positive predictive value and negative predictive value

	Disease	**Healthy**		
Positive diagnosis	True positive rates (a)	False positive rates (b)	Total positive diagnoses (a+b)	*Positive predictive value* – those with positive tests will have the disease a/(a+b)
Negative diagnosis	False negative rates (c)	True negative rates (d)	Total negative diagnoses (c+d)	*Negative predictive value* – those with negative tests will not have the disease d/(c+d)
	Total disease cases (a+c)	Total healthy cases (b+d)	Total number of cases (a+b+c+d)	
	Sensitivity – those with the disease test positive a/(a + c)	*Specificity* – those without the disease test negative d/(b + d)		

Overall predictiveness of a given test result can be summarised as a **likelihood ratio.**

Likelihood ratio positive (LR+): a diseased individual will correctly get a positive ratio (compared to healthy individuals)

$$Likelihood\ ratio\ positive\ (LR+) = \frac{Sensitivity}{(1-specificity)}$$

Likelihood ratio negative (LR-): a healthy individual will correctly get a negative test (compared to diseased individuals)

$$Likelihood\ ratio\ negative\ (LR-) = \frac{(1-specificity)}{Sensitivity}$$

The further away a likelihood ratio is from 1, the stronger the evidence for the presence or absence of disease.

Pre-test probability: number of cases in the population at a specific or time interval (prevalence).

Post-test probability: proportion of patients testing positive who truly have the disease.

Fagan's nomogram[15] links pre-test and post-test probabilities with the likelihood ratios and the usefulness of a diagnostic test.

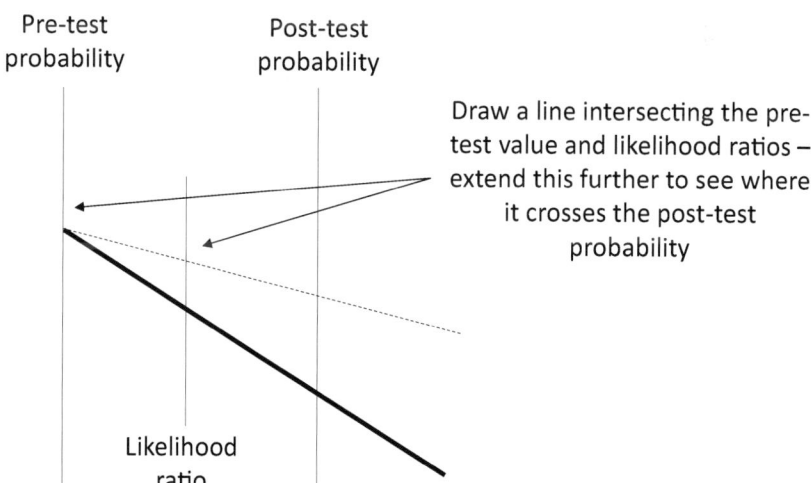

Figure 10.6 How to read a Fagan nomogram

Receiver operating characteristic (ROC) curves compare specificities and sensitivities of tests[16]:

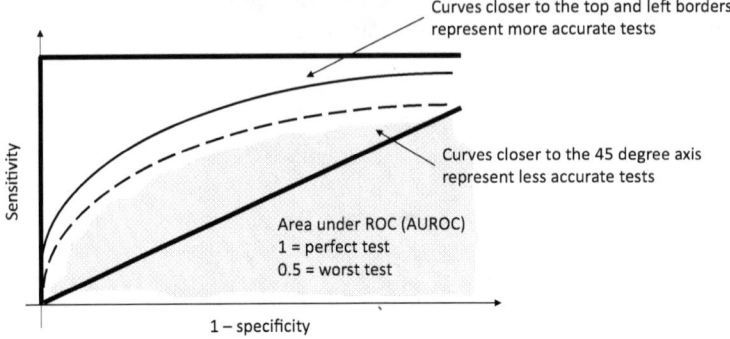

Figure 10.7 Components of a receiver operating curve (ROC)

Kaplan-Meier curves plot survival probability over time and can be useful in cohort and experimental studies. **Median survival** (survival probability of 0.5) can be used to compare different populations and help understand risk.[17]

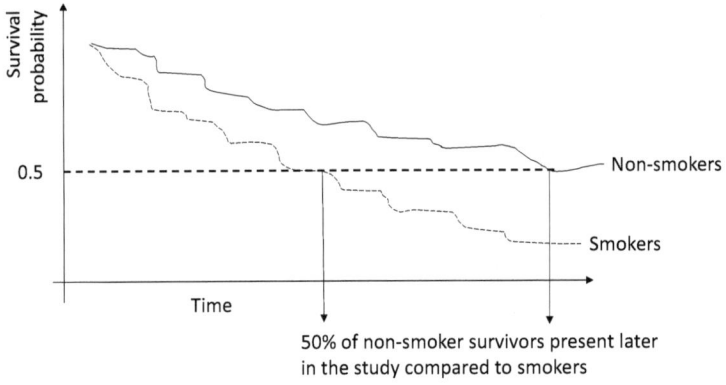

Figure 10.8 Example of a Kaplan-Meier curve

Measures of treatment impact[18]:

Table 10.11 and 10.12 Measures of treatment impact

	Outcome	
	Yes	*No*
Experimental group	A	b
Control group	C	d
Experimental event rate (EER)	Probability of an event occurring in the experimental group.	a/(a+b)

Control event rate (CER)	Probability of an event occurring in the control group.	c/(c+d)
Experimental odds	Chance of an event versus chance of a non-event in an experimental group.	a/b
Control odds	Chance of an event versus chance of a non-event in a control group.	c/d
Odds ratio	Compares experimental and control odds.	(a*d)/(b*c)
Relative risk (RR)	Compares the probability of an outcome in experimental and control groups.	EER/CER
Absolute risk reduction (ARR)	Absolute difference in risks between experimental and control groups for negative outcomes (benefit increase for positive outcomes).	CER-EER
Relative risk reduction (RRR)	Relative difference in risks between experimental and control groups for negative outcomes (benefit increase for positive outcomes)	1-RR
Number needed to treat (NNT)	Number of patients needed to be treated to produce a positive outcome (or number needed to be harmed for negative outcomes).	1/ARR

Hypothesis testing[19-21]

- **Null hypothesis (H_0):** no significant difference between experimental and control groups, where any observed differences are due to chance and chance alone.
  - *'Experimental drug 41CAYT does not improve depressive symptoms in 17-year-olds'.*
- **Alternative hypotheses (H_1):** significant differences exist between experimental and control groups, not due to chance alone.
  - *'Experimental drug 41CAYT does improve depressive symptoms in 17-year-olds'.*

P-values can help support/refute null hypotheses.

- **P ≤ 0.05:** statistically significant results – reject the null hypothesis and accept alternative ones.
- **P > 0.05:** results due to chance – accept the null hypothesis.

Statistical inference involves **generalising** sample data to target populations. **Standard errors** can estimate how representative a sample is of its target population and its generalisability.

Calculating standard error of the mean example:

A psychiatrist has been looking into the weight gain of working-age patients diagnosed with schizophrenia on different antipsychotics. The psychiatrist collects data from a random sample of 50 patients on risperidone and 44 patients on olanzapine and calculates the mean weight gain and standard deviation.

Table 10.13

	Number of patients	Mean weight gain (kg)	Standard deviation (kg)
Risperidone	50	3.5	1.2
Olanzapine	44	4.0	2.5

Standard error (SE) = sample standard deviation/√(sample size)
Risperidone: $1.2/\sqrt{50} = 0.17$
Olanzapine: $2.5/\sqrt{44} = 0.38$

The higher standard error for the olanzapine sample suggests it may be less representative of the population than the risperidone sample.

Confidence intervals provide a range of values likely to include the population value with a defined level of assurance.

Confidence intervals can be used in conjunction with P-values to determine statistical significance:

- If $p \leq 0.05$, confidence intervals should *not* contain 0, as there should be a statistical difference between groups.
- If $p > 0.05$, confidence intervals should contain 0, as there isn't a statistical difference.

Incorrectly accepting alternative hypotheses when the null hypothesis is true can lead to **type 1 errors**, and incorrectly accepting the null hypothesis can lead to **type 2 errors**. A **powerful** study has **larger sample sizes** and **lower propensity for type 2 errors**.

Types of data distribution[22]:

- **Parametric data:** continuous, normally distributed.
- **Non-parametric data:** discrete, non-normally distributed or distribution unknown.

Quick facts about the normal distribution:

- Things like **height** and **weight** are normally distributed in a population.
- Most individuals are clustered around the mean value **with few individuals at the extreme ends**.
- In normally distributed data, the **mean = mode = median**.
- **68%** of data values lie **1 standard deviation** above and below the mean.
- **95%** of data values lie **2 standard deviations** above and below the mean.
- **99.7%** of data values lie **3 standard deviations** above and below the mean.

Parametric statistical tests[22]:

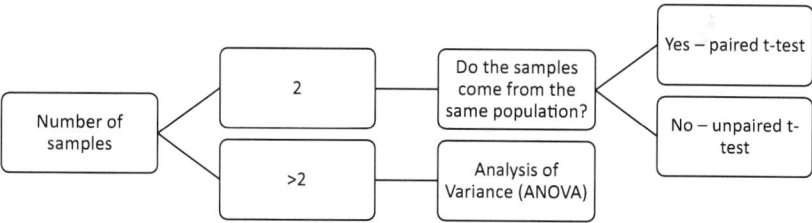

Figure 10.9 Parametric statistical tests

Types of analysis of variance (ANOVA)

- 1-way ANOVA: examining a single input variable and a single outcome.
- 2-way ANOVA: examining 2 input variables and a single outcome.
- ANCOVA: examining a single input variable, a co-variable and a single outcome.
- MANOVA: examining multiple outcomes (can be 1-way or 2-way).
- MANCOVA: includes a co-variable.

Non-parametric statistical tests[22]:

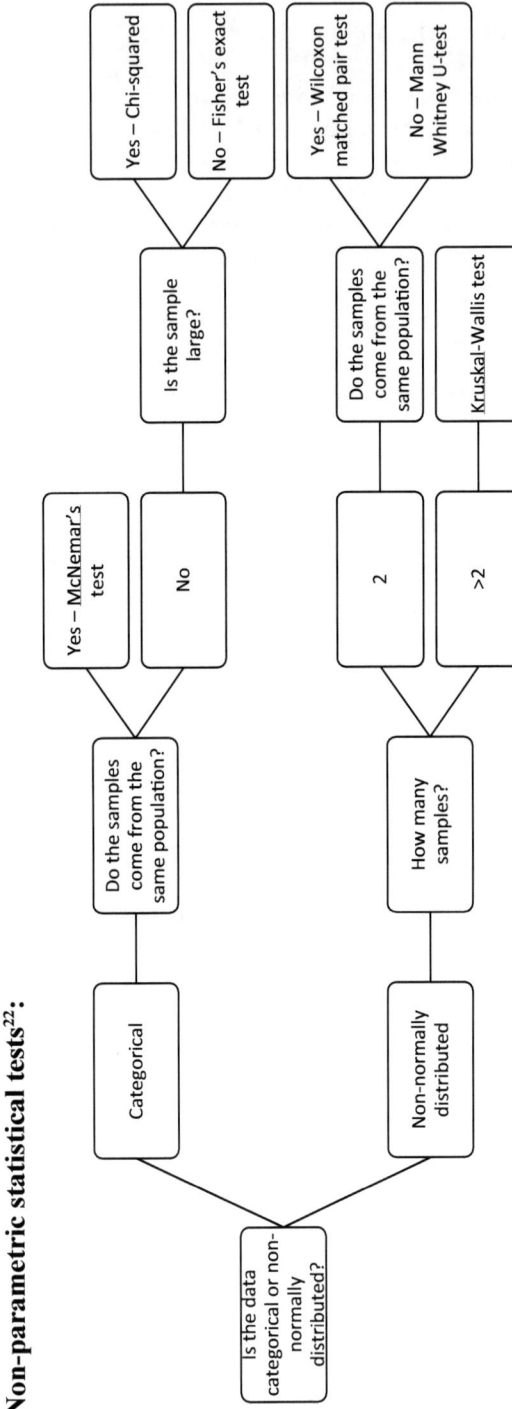

Figure 10.10 Non-parametric statistical tests

Correlation and causality[23]

- **Correlation** ('co-relation') determines whether 2 things are linked, i.e., an individual's height and weight.

  - *Can be graphically represented using **scatter plots***

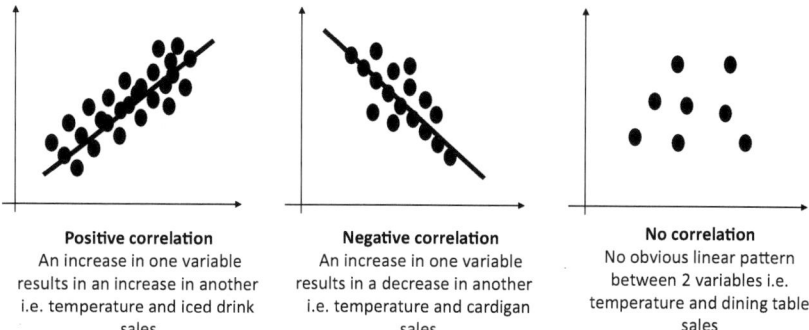

| **Positive correlation** | **Negative correlation** | **No correlation** |
| An increase in one variable results in an increase in another i.e. temperature and iced drink sales | An increase in one variable results in a decrease in another i.e. temperature and cardigan sales | No obvious linear pattern between 2 variables i.e. temperature and dining table sales |

Figure 10.11 Types of scatter plot

- *Quantified using **correlation coefficients***

Pearson correlation coefficient for parametric data and **Spearman correlation coefficient** for non-parametric data. Usually yields values between **-1 and +1** with values closer to 0 representing **weaker correlations**.

- **Causality** establishes whether one event (cause) leads to another (effect), i.e., umbrella use due to rainy weather.

  - *Can be mathematically modelled using **regression analysis***

Regression analysis produces an equation that links variables together. Variables that are linearly related, for example, can be calculated as follows:

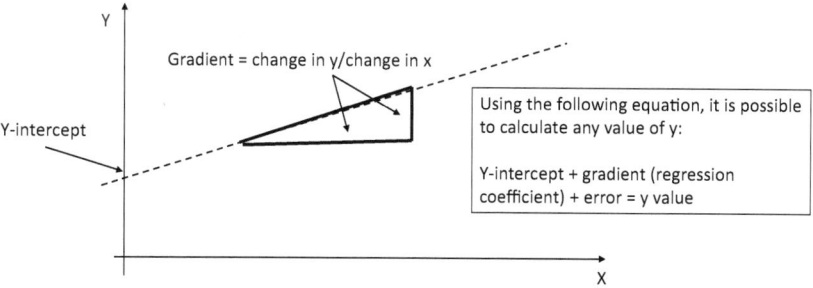

Y

Gradient = change in y/change in x

Y-intercept

Using the following equation, it is possible to calculate any value of y:

Y-intercept + gradient (regression coefficient) + error = y value

X

Figure 10.12 Linear regression analysis

More complex relationships may exist between **multiple** variables or **logistical** ones that follow a **non-linear pattern**.

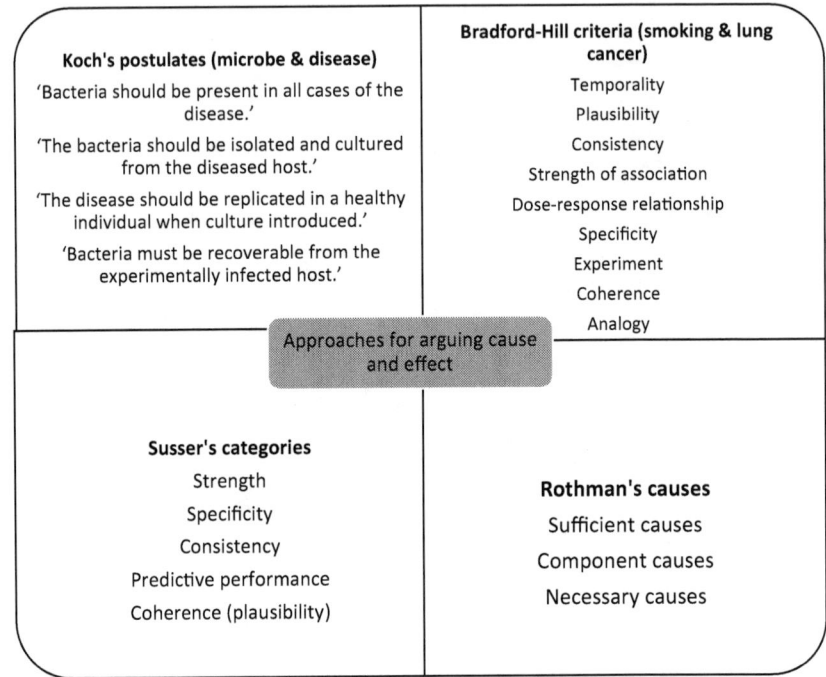

Koch's postulates (microbe & disease)

'Bacteria should be present in all cases of the disease.'

'The bacteria should be isolated and cultured from the diseased host.'

'The disease should be replicated in a healthy individual when culture introduced.'

'Bacteria must be recoverable from the experimentally infected host.'

Bradford-Hill criteria (smoking & lung cancer)

Temporality
Plausibility
Consistency
Strength of association
Dose-response relationship
Specificity
Experiment
Coherence
Analogy

Approaches for arguing cause and effect

Susser's categories

Strength
Specificity
Consistency
Predictive performance
Coherence (plausibility)

Rothman's causes

Sufficient causes
Component causes
Necessary causes

Figure 10.13 Approaches for arguing cause and effect

Confounding – when determining a cause/effect relationship, it is important to limit the impact of other 'confounding' variables. This can be done through:

- **Restriction** (setting inclusion and exclusion criteria).
- **Matching** (distributing variables evenly amongst different study groups).
- Adjusting for variables using **stratification, minimisation** or **multivariable regression models**.

Intention to treat analysis ('once randomised, always analysed')[24]

Ways of handling missing data:

1. Exclude all individuals with incomplete data (**complete case analysis**).
2. Carry forward the last available observation (**LOCF**).
3. Use **worst, average** or **best** data values available.
4. Employ **multiple imputation**.

Meta-analyses improve the power and robustness of research and gather information from all existing studies in an area. **Forest** and **Galbraith plots** display the heterogeneity between studies:

Forest plots[25]:

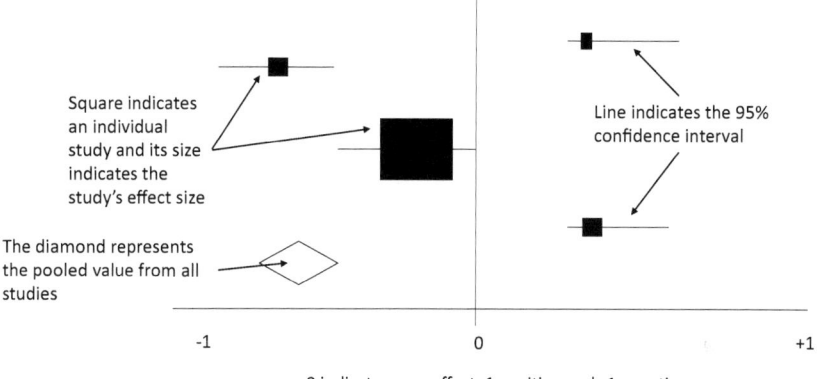

Figure 10.14 Components of a Forest plot

Galbraith plots[26]:

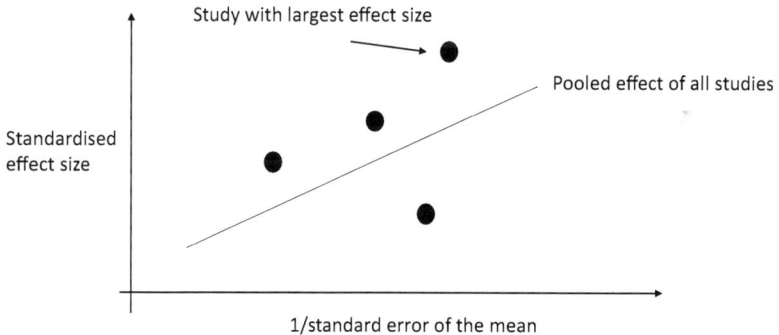

Figure 10.15 Features of a Galbraith plot

The **chi-squared** test can also be used to delineate discrepancies between different studies and the variation between expected and observed outcomes. It is calculated from the sum of (observed frequency − expected frequency) squared divided by the expected frequency.[27]

Key terms in epidemiology:

Prevalence (existing cases)

Point prevalence:
number of cases in a specific population at a particular point in time
／ total population at the same point in time

Period prevalence:
number of cases in a specific population in a defined time period
／ total population in the same time period

Incidence (new cases)

Cumulative incidence (incidence proportion):
number of new cases in a specific population in a defined time period
／ population at the start of the time period

Incidence rate:
number of new cases in a specific population in a defined time period
／ at risk time period

Prevalence =
incidence x duration

Recovered cases

Mortality (deaths)

- Deaths occurring over a particular time period/within a population.
- Can be crude or cause-specific and age specific (infant mortality for example).
- Age adjusted mortality rates eliminate the impact of different age distributions in different populations.
- Standardised mortality ratios (SMR) can be calculated using:

observed number of deaths
／ expected number of deaths

Worked example

An outpatient clinic with a population of 9090 patients wanted to look into the rates of treatment-resistant depression. They collected the following data:

Year	Number of patients with TRD	Total number of clinic patients
2021	1200	6000
2022	1490	9090

Assuming no recoveries or deaths:

Point prevalence in 2021:
1200/6000 = 0.2 (20%)

Cumulative incidence from 2021 to 2022:
(1490 − 1200)/6000 = 290/6000 = 0.048333 (4.83%)

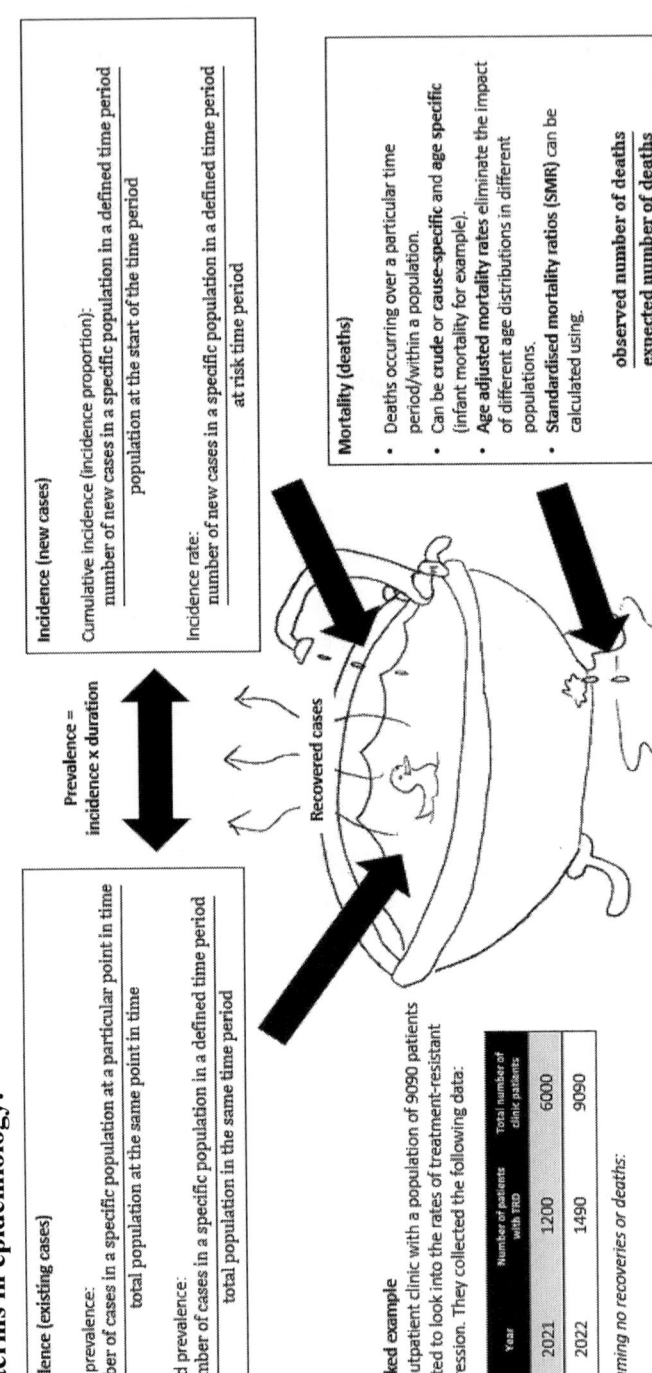

THE EPIDEMIOLOGIST'S BATHTUB (ADAPTED FROM INCIDENCE VS PREVALENCE AND THE EPIDEMIOLOGIST'S BATHTUB | HSC PUBLIC HEALTH AGENCY (HSCNI.NET))

Figure 10.16 The epidemiologist's bathtub[28]

Basic health economics[29]:

Direct vs indirect costs

- **Direct costs** – derived directly from patient care, i.e., bed linen, patient meals.
- **Indirect costs** – not directly related to patient care, i.e., administrator support, IT services, human resources.

Types of economic evaluation

- **Cost-effectiveness analysis (CEA)** – considers benefits of interventions in terms of non-monetary impacts, i.e., improvement in patient symptoms.

> *Cost-effectiveness acceptability curves compare the cost-effectiveness of different interventions by plotting a stakeholder's willingness to pay against incremental cost-effectiveness ratios (ICERS).*

- **Cost-utility analysis (CUA)** – considers benefits of interventions in terms of QALYs and DALYs (see 'Adjusted life years').
- **Cost-benefit analysis (CBA)** – considers benefits of interventions in terms of monetary impact, i.e., reduced accident and emergency attendances.
- **Cost-minimisation analysis (CMA)** – considers benefits of interventions in terms of cost reduction.

> *Sensitivity analyses assess the rigour of an economic evaluation and involve repeating it under different conditions – can be 1-way (extreme scenario, changing a single parameter), multiway or probabilistic.*

Adjusted life years:

- **Quality-adjusted life years (QALYs)** – quantifies how much additional 'time' of decent quality life a patient may gain from a proposed treatment.
- **Disability-adjusted life years (DALYs)** – quantifies how much 'time' a patient loses from a disease/disability without a proposed treatment.

Other key terms:

- **Opportunity costs** – describes the potential benefits stakeholders lose out on when choosing an intervention over another.
- **Discounting** – adjusting for costs occurring at different points in time, i.e., initial start-up costs for a new building 'vs' ongoing rent and bills.
    - *Generally, future costs are given less weight than initial*

Qualitative methods[30,31]

Researchers should adopt **phenomenological approaches** and focus on acquiring '**meaning**' (people's lived experiences).

Methods for collecting data:

- **Surveys** and **questionnaires**.
- **Focus groups** – researchers sparking conversation amongst groups of subjects.
- **Structured interviews** – researchers conversing with individual subjects.
- **Ethnography** – researchers immersing themselves in systems and observing subjects.

Methods for analysing data:

> Data should be **grounded** in subjects' experiences and **inductive** (gathered data used to generate ideas rather than to prove or disprove predefined ideas; '**deductive**').

Process of data analysis in qualitative research:

1. Organise data, i.e., transcripts from interviews, field notes, etc.
2. Review data to identify ideas (**content analysis**).
3. Categorise ideas with 'codes' using clearly defined rules.
4. Regularly review and redefine codes (**constant comparison**).
5. Recognise when no new information emerges (**data saturation**).
6. Link codes with overarching themes (**thematic analysis**).

Methods for data validation:

1. **Triangulation:** multiple researchers, research methodologies and subjects employed to address the same clinical question.
2. **Member checking:** subjects reviewing data prior to analysis to ensure it is accurate and resonates with their experiences.

Methods for minimising bias:

1. **Reflexivity:** researchers considering their own biases and their impact on the research process.
2. **Bracketing:** researchers suspending their biases during the research process.

Guideline and protocol development[32–34]

Commonly used guidelines:

- Scottish Intercollegiate Guidelines Network (SIGN) guidelines.
- NICE (National Institute of Health and Clinical Excellence).

Process for developing guidelines:

1. Identify a guideline development group (GDG).
2. Declare any conflict of interests.
3. Perform literature review and identify clinical question.
4. Review evidence.
5. Make recommendations and draft guidelines.
6. Perform external consultations.
7. Revise guidelines.
8. Obtain external endorsement prior to publication.
9. Distribute and apply guidelines.
10. Update accordingly.

Table 10.14 Advantages and limitations of clinical guidelines

Advantages of guidelines	Limitations of guidelines
• Improve clinical practice. • Reduce variation in practice. • Promote evidence-based practices. • Promote cost-effective measures.	• Unavailability at point of care. • Length of time taken to create. • May not translate to local settings. • Limited patient involvement.

Critical appraisal

Points to consider when reviewing and appraising studies

- *How did you come across the paper? What database did you use? What search strategies did you adopt? What were the inclusion and exclusion criteria? Did you consider publication bias?*
- *What was the clinical question? What were the hypotheses?*
- *What type of study was used and what are its limitations? How was the sample chosen? How did the researchers reduce bias? Were any tools used, and was sensitivity/specificity considered?*
- *What were the results? How were they presented? Would you consider them accurate, precise and valid? Were they qualitative or quantitative? If quantitative, did the authors make use of statistical tests? Were the authors trying to prove causality?*
- *What were the author's analyses? What were their strengths and weaknesses? Have they suggested any recommendations moving forward?*

Helpful tools for appraising studies:

- Quality of Reporting of Meta-Analyses (QUORUM) – can assist in the appraisal of meta-analyses.
- Consolidated Standards of Reporting Trials (CONSORT) – helpful in ascertaining the standardisation and reproducibility of randomised controlled trials.
- Standards for Reporting Studies of Diagnostic Accuracy (STARD) – checklist to assess the quality of studies investigating diagnostic accuracy.
- Critical Appraisal Skills Programme (CASP) – can be used for journal club presentations.

Critical appraisal can be implemented outside exam settings too! For example:

- Applying evidence to clinical practice.

  - *Providing information to patients to enable them to make full and informed decisions*

- Journal club presentations and other workplace-based assessments.
- Clinical governance.
- Audits and quality improvement projects (Plan, Do, Study, Act).

References

1. Sackett DL. Evidence-based medicine. Semin Perinatol. 1997;21(1):3–5. doi: 10.1016/s0146-0005(97)80013-4.
2. https://libguides.winona.edu/ebptoolkit/ClinicalQ#:~:text=Background%20questions%20ask%20for%20general%20knowledge%20about%20a,specific%20knowledge%20to%20inform%20clinical%20decisions%20or%20actions. Accessed 11/22.
3. https://onlinenursing.duq.edu/blog/formulating-a-picot-question/ Accessed 11/22.
4. McCombes S. Types of research designs compared | Guide & examples. *Scribbr*, 3 January 2023, www.scribbr.com/methodology/types-of-research/ Accessed 11/22
5. Resources for Evidence-Based Practice: The 6S Pyramid. *Secondary Resources for Evidence-Based Practice: The 6S Pyramid*, 2016. http://hsl.mcmaster.libguides.com/ebm
6. www.nice.org.uk/process/pmg20/chapter/identifying-the-evidence-literature-searching-and-evidence-submission Accessed 11/22.
7. Lefebvre C, Glanville J, Briscoe S, et al. Chapter 4: Searching for and selecting studies. In Higgins JPT, Thomas J, Cumpston M et al. (eds). *Cochrane Handbook for Systematic Reviews of Interventions Version 6.2 (updated February 2021)*. London: Cochrane, 2021.
8. Rosenthal R., The file drawer problem and tolerance for null results. Psychol Bull. 1979; 86: 638–641.
9. Asiamah N., et al. General, target and accessible population: Demystifying the concepts for effective sampling. Qual Rep. 2017; 22(6): 1607–1622.
10. McCombes S. Sampling methods | types, techniques & examples. *Scribbr*, 27 March 2023. www.scribbr.com/methodology/sampling-methods

11. Middleton F. Reliability vs. validity in research | difference, types and examples. *Scribbr*, 30 January 2023. www.scribbr.com/methodology/reliability-vs-validity/ Accessed 11/22.

12. GPossall N, Gossall G. *The doctor's guide to critical appraisal*, 5th edition, 2020. Knutsford, UK: Pastest.

13. White S. *Basic & Clinical Biostatistics*, 5th edition (A& L Lange series). London: McGraw Hill, 2019.

14. www.healthknowledge.org.uk/e-learning/statistical-methods/specialists/diagnostic-tests Accessed 11/22.

15. Akobeng AK. Understanding diagnostic tests 2: Likelihood ratios, pre- and post-test probabilities and their use in clinical practice. Acta Paediatr. 2007;96(4):487–491. doi: 10.1111/j.1651-2227.2006.00179.x

16. Park SH, Goo JM, Jo CH. Receiver operating characteristic (ROC) curve: Practical review for radiologists. Korean J Radiol. 2004;5(1):11–18. doi: 10.3348/kjr.2004.5.1.11

17. https://towardsdatascience.com/kaplan-meier-curves-c5768e349479 Accessed 11/22

18. Irwig L, Irwig J, Trevena L, et al. Chapter 18, Relative risk, relative and absolute risk reduction, number needed to treat and confidence intervals. In *Smart Health Choices: Making Sense of Health Advice*. London: Hammersmith Press, 2008. www.ncbi.nlm.nih.gov/books/NBK63647/

19. Bevans, R. Hypothesis testing | A step-by-step guide with easy examples. *Scribbr*, 7 December 2022. www.scribbr.com/statistics/hypothesis-testing/

20. Bhandari, P. What is standard error? | How to calculate (Guide with examples). *Scribbr*, 19 December 2022. www.scribbr.com/statistics/standard-error/

21. O'Brien SF, Yi QL. How do I interpret a confidence interval? Transfusion. 2016;56(7):1680–1683. doi: 10.1111/trf.13635.

22. Bevans, R. Choosing the right statistical test | Types & examples. *Scribbr*, 5 December 2022. www.scribbr.com/statistics/statistical-tests/

23. www.khanacademy.org/test-prep/praxis-math/praxis-math-lessons/gtp – praxis-math – lessons – statistics-and-probability/a/gtp – praxis-math – article – correlation-and-causation – lesson Accessed 11/23

24. Sedgwick P. What is intention to treat analysis? BMJ 2013; 346:f3662. doi:10.1136/bmj.f3662

25. https://s4be.cochrane.org/blog/2016/07/11/tutorial-read-forest-plot/ Accessed 11/22

26. www.erim.eur.nl/research-support/meta-essentials/user-manual/work-with-the-workbooks/publication-bias-analysis-sheet/galbraith-plot/ Accessed 11/22

27. Turney, S. Chi-Square (X^2) Tests | types, formula & examples. *Scribbr*. 10 November 2022 www.scribbr.com/statistics/chi-square-tests/

28. Incidence vs prevalence and the epidemiologist's bathtub | HSC Public Health Agency, hscni.net Accessed 11/22

29. Kernick DP. Introduction to health economics for the medical practitioner. Postgrad Med J. 2003;79:147–150.

30. Bhandari, P. What is qualitative research? | Methods & examples. *Scribbr*, 30 January 2023. www.scribbr.com/methodology/qualitative-research/

31. Hennink et al. *Qualitative research methods*. London: Sage publications, 2020.

32. NIPCE | The National Institute for Health and Care Excellence, https://www.nice.org.uk/guidance/ Accessed 11/22

33. www.sign.ac.uk/our-guidelines/ Accessed 11/22.

34. Shekelle. Developing guidelines. BMJ 1999;318:593

Index

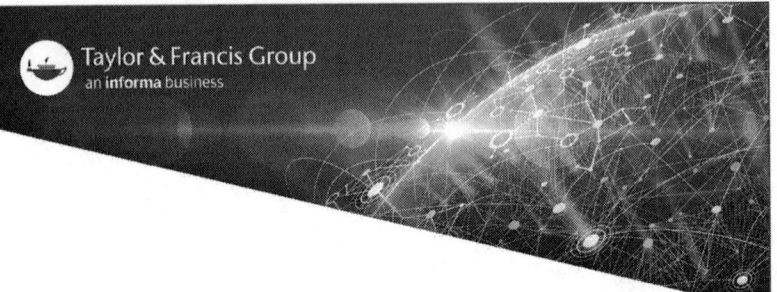
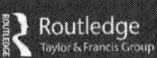
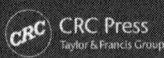